THE SPIRIT CODE
Christ-Centered Energy Healing

Self-Sabotage
Manual

ISBN:
9781794573215

Front cover photograph by Daniel Hopkins
Visit danielhopkins.com

Table of Contents

Introduction

Disclaimer: Your results may vary. This is not intended to replace or substitute conventional medical care, or encourage its abandonment. This program does not guarantee any specific results. Your results are based off of God's will, your readiness, the atonement and long-term dedication towards your personal development. Please take full responsibility for your results and your own health and well-being.

This manual is a part of The Spirit Code's Christ-Centered Energy Healing program. This program is designed for those seeking the "next step" in energy healing. In this manual we explore how to shift your interpretation of the past, live mindfully in the present and shift your expectations for the future while releasing negative energy. This is the "life coaching" portion of our program combined with energy releases to assist in lifestyle changes. This manual also includes the Emotional Freedom Technique (EFT), also known as "tapping," which assists the body in rebalancing hormones.

Self-sabotage is a negative lifestyle pattern currently being engaged in and is, therefore, a "living energy." Within the energy healing world, it is a common practice to "release" negative energy; however, **releasing <u>live</u> negative energy will not achieve long-lasting successful results until an internal change occurs. This is because the energy will be recreated as we fall into the same patterns that created the energy in the first place.** These steps are designated to be done interactively for longer lasting change.

When beginning an internal change and shifting a lifestyle pattern, you are never alone. Ask for God's healing love to come into your heart and mind; to become humble, teachable and accountable. Although a self-sabotaging lifestyle is the most difficult energy to change; it is also the most rewarding. Life does not end at death; our thoughts, emotions, addictions, patterns and memories go with us into the spirit world. This life is an opportunity to grow, heal, nurture and progress. If this self-sabotage pattern doesn't change **now**, it will continue to affect spiritual progression, even past this mortal life. **Eternal happiness is not offered to us, it is created within us.**

Energy is all around; you are energy and you attract more energy with every experience you have. There are positive and negative forms of energy that are influential on the spirit, mind, body and energy fields. When we hold onto negative energy, our health can suffer greatly as we tend to create a lifestyle that revolves around negativity. Breaking this lifestyle cannot be done for you by someone else, nor can it be done alone either. Creating change requires new understandings of the past so you can reflect upon the most traumatic events and feel compassion and forgiveness for yourself and all others involved. **Healing also requires action** – a conscious commitment to follow through with changes to your daily habits and patterns that formed the negative lifestyle. In many circumstances, our lifestyles have been deeply embedded within us over the course of decades. We cannot emphasize enough how important it is to take action with a strong commitment to uproot the current lifestyle and lay a new foundation for healthy roots to grow. All energy can be self-created, inherited, absorbed, living or created by another to intentionally inflict harm. Being aware of the origination is helpful, but not necessary unless it's living/active.

Self-Sabotage leads us into traps. You may have heard the phrase, "We work jobs we hate, to buy stuff we don't need to fill up a house we cannot afford." Additionally, we seek connection and love, but push people away or build up walls and barriers for protection to keep others out, and then experience loneliness and disconnection in relationships. As a result, we feel sick, overweight, addicted, angry, victimized and completely alone in a world full of opportunities and people. When physical or mental symptoms present themselves; the body is communicating that there is a problem. It's time to begin listening, accepting accountability and making necessary changes.

This manual is broken down into a step by step program to break free from self-sabotage. There are 12 steps to this program, however there's a master's program with an additional 4 steps for those seeking further development once mastering this program. These steps are meant to be taught and worked through with an energy healer. This program is NOT successful when done alone and simply by reading the manual. The assignments and further energy work must be completed with another person to produce results. It is recommended to use one step per session for greater success and completing the dark energy releases must be completed before reaching step 11 or the full release will not be successful. The same goes for sensory and trauma energies. However, everyone is at a different phase of their healing journey, so some steps can be condensed and spirit to spirit communication may also increase the results for those a level 700 and beyond.

We use muscle testing to properly communicate with the body the "cause" of each symptom, then follow through with complete healing in the spirit, mind and body. Always test your client and tailor the program based upon their needs. It is critical that each client commits to completing all of the self-sabotage steps. It is also critical to do an energy release with each step as found in the Spirit Code program. Our program is best done interactively, as true change is not done for others, rather it is a journey taken together. If your client has any "processing," quickly clean up until all energetic wounds are healed, so they are not left with exhaustion. There should be no processing when done properly. Always feel free to contact us for further guidance. We also offer classes on our website - spiritcode.net.

The goals of this program include, but are not limited to:

- Release the destructive bonds of the past through energy work.
- Heal the spirit, mind, and body.
- Practice personal development and manifest the life you desire by setting the course for your life and taking action steps.

- Coming to peace with your past.
- Breaking through your walls and barriers.
- Recognize what mistakes are producing undesirable results and what areas need improvement.
- Break free of the victim cycle.
- Become the conscious creator of your own life.
- Offer compassion for those you have harmed and those who harmed you.
- Experience self-love, life affirming self-talk, and practice self-care.
- Take responsibility for your life and change your course.
- Repent: experience the healing power of the atonement and forgive yourself.
- To fully internalize that this life is about learning and progressing therefore creating a safe space for healing.
- Reflect upon the past and feel love /forgiveness.
- See the future differently, because your interpretation of the past brings peace.
- Find gratitude for the life you are living.
- Balance the hormone production in your body through EFT.
- Begin shifting thought patterns in the manner Jesus Christ has taught, so you do not repeat past mistakes.
- Become prepared to live the higher law of Moses in preparation for the second coming of Jesus Christ.
- To walk the streets of New Jerusalem and share your emotions, thoughts and energy with all others, while radiating complete Christ-like love, even to those who were once considered your enemy.

The most effective way to heal emotionally, spiritually, mentally and physically is by incorporating the higher law of Moses and the teachings of Jesus Christ into your life. When you focus on the atonement and inquire of God on how to heal for the purpose of Godly service, you can receive guidance and personal revelation geared specifically towards you. All healing comes from Christ, so please take the time to consider His ability and offer gratitude for His gift of healing. We can repay Him by serving our fellow brothers and sisters.

Matthew 25: 31-40 (KJV)

31 When the Son of man shall come in his glory, and all the holy angels with him, then shall he sit upon the throne of his glory:
32 And before him shall be gathered all nations: and he shall separate them one from another, as a shepherd divideth his sheep from the goats:
33 And he shall set the sheep on his right hand, but the goats on the left.
34 Then shall the King say unto them on his right hand, Come, ye blessed of my Father, inherit the kingdom prepared for you from the foundation of the world:
35 For I was an hungered, and ye gave me meat: I was thirsty, and ye gave me drink: I was a stranger, and ye took me in:
36 Naked, and ye clothed me: I was sick, and ye visited me: I was in prison, and ye came unto me.

37 Then shall the righteous answer him, saying, Lord, when saw we thee an hungered, and fed thee? or thirsty, and gave thee drink?

38 When saw we thee a stranger, and took thee in? or naked, and clothed thee?

39 Or when saw we thee sick, or in prison, and came unto thee?

40 And the King shall answer and say unto them, Verily I say unto you, Inasmuch as ye have done it unto one of the least of these my brethren, ye have done it unto me."

Within this manual we refer to the "How to Create a Compound" manual and "The Spirit Code Healing Program." For more information regarding the manual and program visit Spiritcode.net or contact us at thespiritcode@gmail.com. Our entire program consists of intuitive healing, muscle testing, visualizations, energy releases, dark curse removal, EFT-tapping, life coaching, self-sabotage work, energetic compounds, and atonement steps. This "self-sabotage" section is a critical component, but only a fraction of the entire program. We work in conjunction with God's creations as we rely upon the angels and the earth's healing energy. We work on healing the spirit first, then the mind and then the body. Healing is not instant, nor is it simple. We have complex bodies which require thorough methods of healing.

In this manual we make references to "rebellious spirits" or "the rebellion." This is a term offered to all spirits who have not chosen to follow God and are, therefore, rebelling. This term encompasses all different types of spirits. When we clear our space of all negative influences; it is critical to include all of the rebellious spirits and their influences as well.

Some of the energetic forms of influence that rebellious spirits exercise over mortals are called "Self-Destructive Tools of Dark Influences" (SDT) and "Mind Subconscious Suggestions" (MSS). The SDT encompass 28 types of energies which include curses and sabotages. The MSS comprise of 67 types which are given as thoughts or images and are presented to a person's mind. They include post-hypnotic suggestions, subliminal messages, despair anchors, broadcast messages and images. The SDT and MSS are also commonly used by mortals simply by wishing ill intent upon another. Remember, our thoughts and intentions are powerful and they literally can cause a great amount of destruction in others. Steps to remove the rebellious spirits and their influences are included in the Appendix.

We have been given the Spirit Code program through personal revelation for the purpose of taking energy work to the next level and prepare ourselves for the second coming of Christ. This includes physical healing as well as emotional and spiritual healing. We are here to stretch forth our hands and offer assistance to our brothers and sisters as we are all equals experiencing life together. We have been given a gift and we wish to share this gift with others. Let's take this journey together towards healing from self-sabotage, so we may fully live our callings as co-creators with our Heavenly Father. You are not alone! You are loved!

Self-Sabotage
Step One

"God cares alot **more** about who we are and who we are becoming than about who we once were" - Dale A Renlund

Clear Your Space

Test your client to see if these steps need to be completed before continuing. These steps are found in the Appendix. Always begin your appointments by checking for "attacks."

1. Begin by clearing the space and removing all dark influences/rebellious spirits
2. Remove Self-Destructive Tools of Dark Influences
3. Remove Mind Subconscious suggestions
4. Remove Intimidation Energy
5. Ask for shields of protection

~~~~~~

Mall Mapping

In order to properly align your current reality with your desired results, you must first find your starting point and plan a route to naturally reach your destination. This is similar to mall mapping. Example – you need a classy dress for a business event, so you go shopping at the mall. Two instances will produce two very different results. The mall will remain the same; the selection will also; however, your experience and the results will prove how crucial personal development work truly is.

Scenario one: You have put off this purchase for a few months and now the event is upon you. You are feeling rushed and only have one day to shop for the event. You are having a rough day, feeling fat, drained, and grouchy with very little money in your account. You don't know what you want to buy or what store to shop at, but you want it to be affordable and make you feel amazing. You wander around the mall searching in all the wrong places. You have never been to this mall, making it hard to find your favorite stores. You do find a few comparable options, but everything you try on is too youthful, too mature, too snug or too loose. While you are trying on clothes the thoughts running through your head are: I am so fat, I look awful in this, I need to lose weight, I hate shopping, and my boss is going to be embarrassed of me. This makes you even more frustrated as the event is approaching soon. So you settle on something way out of your price range and put it on a credit card. The dress isn't right for your personality, the whole evening you are miserable due to a wardrobe malfunction. You regret your purchase and wish you could have a "do-over", but there's a no-refund policy at the store. You wind up depressed with a load of regret.

Scenario two: You prepare yourself in advance and save up your money. You shop around online for sales and set aside a day for this shopping trip. You know you want a long red dress that's modest with an empire waist. You saw an ad online for the perfect dress at your favorite store at the local mall, it's even on sale. You take care of yourself by eating, and getting plenty of rest before shopping. You walk into the mall with your head held high feeling happy and the thoughts in your head are: what a beautiful day to be alive, I love myself; I'm so excited to show off my inner beauty with this elegant red classy dress. When you enter the mall you first find the mall map that says YOU ARE HERE with a big red X. You look for your desired store on the map and plan a simple route to get there. You begin on your journey and naturally reach your destination. Upon entering the store, you go straight to the map and find the section with formal wear. Again you easily plan a course to the proper section. You easily find the dress you want, at the price you can afford, and feel great when trying it on. Your thoughts are, what a beautiful dress, I can wear this anywhere and dress it up or down, it's even on clearance, I'm so grateful and I feel beautiful. You feel great about your purchase and leave the store rejuvenated. The event flows smoothly and you even have a chance at a promotion. You love this dress so much and it's perfect for many other events.

Moral of the story: This life you are leading is the creation of your choices. Once you know what you want and how to align your current reality with your dreams, you will naturally reach your destination. However the opposite is also true; you can find yourself stranded in life with no clear direction and experiencing misery.

How many times have you found yourself just living day to day with no real clarity or happiness? Have you ever looked around at your life and wanted a do-over? Have you watched others who are succeeding and wished you could have even a small portion of their success? Do you know what you want out of life? Do you know how to accomplish your goals or dreams? Do you keep sabotaging your progress?

This is your life, your only chance to be you and to experience this very moment. Do you want to create something new? Do you want new results? Do you want to break free of the limiting beliefs, the faulty self-talk, the faulty core-beliefs, the self-sabotage and all your limitations? Do you desire different results than what you are experiencing?

We will explore this throughout the next 12 steps of this program to find your starting point, where you are going and how to align your current reality with your desired results to naturally manifest your true purpose. You can consciously create and fulfill your higher purpose and align your will with God's will, naturally by living your purpose. Let's begin this journey together. When checking your own "mall map" we need to find your starting point.

You Are Here ✕

Where are you now, where are you going and how will you get there? Let's take a journey through a simple visualization to honestly examine the reality of your current lifestyle.

Visualization: Close your eyes and I want you to visualize yourself in your safe space – relaxing in your home or upon the beach or hiking the mountains. Wherever you choose, you are alone and free to experience this event excluding ALL judgment from others. There are no distractions, no electronics and no clocks. There is only the sound of silence. I want you to listen inward to your thoughts that are filled with faulty self-talk, contention with family members and complaints in all areas of your life; including health, relationships and personal frustrations. I want you to be completely honest with yourself and how you truly feel about your past and the world around you, but most importantly how you feel about yourself and your current life. Nobody is involved in this visualization so you are free to experience your life in a space of complete honesty.

In this safe space, I want you to look up and see that your life is playing on a screen in front of you, with you as the only viewer. The video starts with your early childhood, playing out all the trials and blessings alike. The movie speeds up and jumps a few years to your youth where you are developing your personality and dreams for your future. Skipping ahead again, go to the first time you moved away from your parents to live on your own. Before you know it, the video is playing your current reality; including your current choices, mindset, belief system, health issues, mental state and family life. Again the film skips ahead one year as a natural progression of these belief systems and your current path in life. What is playing on the film and what does your life look like? Ask yourself these questions:

1. In this year have you played the victim role?
2. How have your patterns or faulty thought processes influenced your life and those around you?

Focus back on the movie and again the film skips ahead; this time 5 years go by in front of your eyes. Time tends to solidify our thought patterns and emotional responses so your patterns are now becoming a way of life. I want you to honestly watch this film and witness where your life is taking you in your current patterns. What do you see? How has your life progressed over these 5 years? Ask yourself these questions:

1. Are you happy with the path that your life has taken?
2. Are you experiencing any regret?
3. How do you feel about yourself?

Once again focus upon the movie as 5 more years fly by. As you can imagine, each thought has turned into words, beliefs, unhappiness, illness, contention, rejection, etc. However it looks in your life, let it play out. These thoughts filled up a whole day, which turned into a week, then a month, then a year, then 5 years, and now 10 years. In this space 10 years into your future, you are experiencing an opportunity to honestly look at your life. I want you to see how the thoughts you had many years ago are affecting you as they have become your core belief system. This is how you now view the world and yourself. These years of thinking a certain way have created your natural subconscious emotional reactions that you currently have little control over. As you watch this film of your life 10 years in the future, I want you to honestly look at your life and ask yourself these questions:

1. Are you experiencing the life you desire for yourself and your family in this space?
2. What changes in your life have occurred during these 10 years?
3. Are you experiencing a different result from that which you prefer for your life?
4. Are you living your dreams?

This space that you have placed yourself in, while reviewing scenes from your past has given you a welcomed opportunity to ponder your life and the possibilities laid before you. Allow yourself to relax in this safe space and watch as the film reverses back to the present moment. Open your eyes and take a moment to offer yourself patience, love and acceptance; as this journey is meant to be a learning opportunity where we make mistakes and grow. What a blessing to return to a lifestyle before events solidify your path. We may consciously create a different outcome over the next few weeks by changing a faulty belief system and improving patterns which will also improve the future.

1. Do you have anything you would like to share that you experienced during this visualization?
2. Have you recognized that there may be a problem which needs correcting?
3. Are you ready for the next step?

God never said it would be easy, but he did promise it would be worth it. The purpose of this exercise is to help you to see that a change needs to occur in order to experience the dream you desire for your life. In order to proceed, you must be honest with yourself and willing to humble yourself to God's will. You cannot reach your true desires or potential without effort. There is hope and a solution that we are progressing towards. Remember to be patient with the process and with yourself.

The body is an amazing creation of our Father in Heaven. Our bodies were created perfectly in His image and have the ability to heal themselves. When you experience an injury such as a broken bone, a burn or a cut; your body naturally heals itself over time. If you are experiencing chronic illness with no real solution or understanding of the cause; it is time to open your mind to the possibility that experiences in life that are filled with emotions and traumas could be the cause of your physical symptoms. Stress has the potential to increases cortisol levels. Many people with an excess amount of stress also experience physical symptoms such as ulcers, weight issues or turn to addictions such as smoking or drinking. People who experience anxiety may have panic attacks, or irrational fears of leaving the house. People who struggle with anger management may experience a heart attack early in life or high blood pressure or stroke. These are just examples of how emotions can create physical symptoms. Emotions are automatic responses due to your understanding of the world around you and the core beliefs that have been created due to your past experiences in life. We will discuss this further throughout the manual.

~~~~~~

Wall Removal

Most people place emotional barriers or walls around themselves for protection. This is automatic and created out of pain or heartache for survival, but it also removes the ability to experience true connection. Walls or barriers can be placed around certain body parts, the whole body or between you and others (including God). There is no need to hold onto a wall during your healing journey, in fact, the success of our program relies upon your ability to process the information and make critical changes. Muscle test: is it safe to remove these walls before continuing? For the majority of clients, it is important to communicate with the body that they are no longer in danger and are no longer living in the past and these walls are unnecessary.

Removing one or two walls is a simple process; however, we would like to remove all of the walls, along with the energy that is the hidden factor behind these walls. We will be going through an interactive visualization. Being honest with yourself throughout this process will greatly improve the chances of success. Each wall was created due to an energy. Be sure to remove the energy as well in order for the wall to not be reformed. For non-contracted walls – simply say – I covert all walls into a rainbow which is a promise that I will allow others to love me and I will not block them out again.

Contracted walls:

1. I bring to light all the walls and contracts
2. How many contracted walls do I have?
3. Remove the rebellious spirits and the contracts:
    a. I bring to light the rebellious spirits, the contracts and the portals attached to each wall.
    b. I wash all the contracts with the living waters and with any remaining, I burn them with the light of Christ.
    c. I detach all cords to the contracts and rebellious spirits, cut the cords (or chains) with the Sword of Limited Freedom, release and remove their cords. I ask for the light rod to break any remaining chains.
    d. Offer the rebellious spirit three choices: 1) Repent and become an angel in training 2) Depart by your own free will 3). Or if you choose to remain or attack, I will cast you out.
        i. For any remaining rebellious spirits; in the name of Jesus Christ I command you to depart immediately. I seal any and all associated portals.
4. **Visualization:** I want you to close your eyes and visualize yourself... you are most likely alone. Where are you? Is there a wall or barrier? How tall is it? What does it look like? Maybe you are stranded on an island, maybe you are in an igloo or a tower. Is there a ceiling? Is there a floor? Is there any way out? Describe what you see and how it feels. Do you feel safe leaving this space? Is anyone else in this space with you? This wall

represents all the walls you have created for protection. This space feels safe and has provided you a safe haven for protection. However, God desires that we love one another and He desires us to experience life with others. This place was created due to difficult experiences which have produced painful emotions. God would not tell you or want you to hide away from the world, but there is someone else who would. Ask God to shine a light of truth upon this space to show you what it really looks like. This place was NOT created by God; it was inspired by the adversary. Ask God to show you the true nature of this space and what influences are here. What do you see now? (*Most people see darkness or traps.*) Would you like to continue staying here or do you wish to leave this space and remove these walls so you can find safety in God's light? Would you like to join your family and leave this lonely existence? (*Allow this to flow into a discussion.*)

5. Now it is time to conquer each wall one at a time. Remember this wall is energetic and lives within your mind. So, we can remove it with the mind. Blow it up or convert it into something mild or climb over it. Get creative, there are no restrictions as gravity does not apply, follow your instinct and conquer each wall. You no longer need it, simply remove it how you wish. Or find a way to leave and walk away. God has a much safer space waiting for you where you can experience true connection with your loved ones.

    a. Continue on this step until they have overcome each wall. This may take some time.

6. Heavenly Father offers protection that is love based not fear based. Now it is time to remember gravity only applies to your body. You can go anywhere; you can fly to find your spouse/children/parents/family. These barriers have no hold over you anymore, it is time to leave and you can find safety in the healing light and love of God. If a couple is doing this together, have the wife shine the light of Christ so bright that it shines through the universe. Now have the husband look up to find her. Or have the mother find the children. Focus upon the love and relationship and the travel will occur naturally. Once reunited, the families can experience a deeper connection and be ready to progress in the healing journey. If family is not an option, then simply ask for Heavenly Father or Jesus Christ to shine their light so bright you can see it throughout the universe. Then focus on His love and healing protection. There's no need to search for Him, just focus on Him and you will find yourself in His healing presence. Focus on being in a cloud of white healing light. This space is a whole new version of safety while being free. Now ask Heavenly Father for protection if you are still in need of a boundary with certain people. This will be a loving Godly wall.

7. There is an energy that created each wall or was connected to each contracted wall. Now that you have removed the walls, go through and remove the energies associated with each wall. You can muscle test the amount of time you have to complete the work before the wall is reformed.

Here are some examples of wall removals: "I was in a field of wild flowers surrounded by a forest. I felt safe and secure in this field but could not enter the forest. I was alone but content. It felt vulnerable to leave this place, but I pushed myself out of my comfort zone and pushed through the barrier of trees. I stepped out and when I did so, the trees deflated and the entire place seemed to fall flat to the ground as if I had been in a bubble. At first, I felt vulnerable, but my spouse removed his walls and we embraced each other and we were able to truly become one and experience love in a way I had never experienced before." Another example: "I was in an igloo, it was cold and the opening was smaller than my hand. The entire igloo was as small as a porcupine which means I was small while inside this igloo. The cold was lacking any warmth of love as I was forgotten. I decided I did not want to live that way any longer and so I imagined myself standing tall, as tall as everyone else and breaking free from this cage. I then turned and stomped on the igloo and ran into the open arms of my wife." Another example (a child): "I was in a small room like a bank vault with lead walls so thick not even an atomic bomb could knock them down. My mother came to rescue me and gave me a pep talk about keeping me safe as a family so I'm no longer alone. I trusted her and we opened the door together, but there standing at the door was a guard who attacked us when we tried to leave. I was free to leave after the guard was removed and I joined my family. I felt very alive and grateful to know I can feel safe in healthier ways."

As you can see a wall removal is very specific for each individual. This release will include all walls and the emotions that created the walls. There is no need to address each specific emotion or memory. However, we can recreate walls every time there is conflict, so this may become a common visualization until you learn how to respond more effectively. We can also recreate walls if there is a "living energy," which means a current conflict that is not yet resolved. Once the automatic thought process is reprogrammed in the manner God created, the walls will no longer be recreated.

Vibrations

Vibrations are simply how we measure your body's energy. We are energy. Our entire existence is energy. Our bodies are living organisms. If we are injured, our bodies heal themselves. They were created perfectly by God to survive. Therefore, anything we invite into our bodies – whether it is food or emotions or thoughts, it affects our bodies. When our brains process an event, our automatic emotional response elevates and our glands respond with an increase or decrease in hormones. A simple way to begin your journey of healing is by raising your own vibrations. Higher vibrations offer increased energy flow and healing. Many people suffer with depression and these emotions and thoughts stay with them unless they overcome them through the healing power of Christ.

The purpose of raising our food's vibrations is to increase hydration and proper absorption of nutrition, so we reap the benefits of the foods we eat, which increases our energy and health. Your food and water are processed by many people before it reaches you. The vibrations in your water have the potential to be in the thousands, but by the time it touches your lips it may only be 10. As a result, many people struggle with dehydration. No matter how much water they drink, they simply cannot absorb the nutritional benefits.

We also tend to overeat as we may find ourselves going into the kitchen just wanting something or mindlessly overeating. The food you are ingesting was once growing in the fields under the sun and alive in the soils. So, what's changed from the time it was plucked until the time you fill your plate? If the vibrations decreased significantly, it is a result of the handlers of this food or water in addition to chemicals and processing. We began an experiment in our own kitchen to raise the vibrations of our food and water. We tested the vibrations of the water in a pitcher, the water from the filter, the food in the pantry and the food in the fridge. Then we played soft church hymns in the kitchen continuously while offering positive thoughts to the food and water. We tested the same food and water a few hours later and the results were amazing. The vibrations of the tap water rose from 13 to 360; and the filtered water rose from 47 to 510. The food had similar results. Therefore, a glass of water has the potential to hydrate the body, while the food can be digested and absorbed more efficiently. I have found myself more satisfied with my meals too. When we pray over our meal, we are essentially doing the same thing. I would like to encourage you to look for ways to increase the positive energy in your home. If there's a lot of contention, it will influence your food; so, offer a prayer for your food, play uplifting music in the kitchen and present a healthy environment for your food. Many times, the reason for a food intolerance is an energy or the lack of desire to exist. Sometimes it is the low vibrations of the food source. Water comes from many sources, but in general raising the vibrations of water will increase hydration and decrease food intolerances.

~~~~~~

Assignments

Energy work:

1. Test which dark energy created the wall and <u>do this release today</u>, this is a critical step. If the energy is a living energy, be aware the wall removal may need to be repeated until your client heals fully from the situation they are experiencing.
2. Invite and absorb into the meridian a continuous flow of: God's healing love, sunlight, peace, patience, gentleness and self-love to be continuously invited in for the next 30-90 days and to be distributed throughout the body, mind and soul freely for the purpose of raising vibrations for healing. Test for any additional emotional or spiritual energies from the chart in the Appendix on page 127.
3. Test for any further healing needs such as the heart/spirit in more than one piece, energetic wounds, or if they need a healing compound.
4. Test for types of infections and prepare a treatment plan for future appointments.
5. Test for toxins and prepare a treatment plan for future appointments.
6. Test for any specific food intolerances. This will assist the body in the healing process to offer a healing environment free of complicated digestive issues. The causes will be addressed and removed, but the healing journey takes time and patience. The more you communicate with the body's needs, the more you will experience your desired results.
   a. Ask: Is this good for me?
   b. Does my body want it?
   c. Can I digest it?
   d. Can I absorb it?
   e. Will this harm my body?
   f. Put together a list so the client is gaining the maximum amount of nutrients from their diet for the healing process. This will only be a temporary diet until the "cause" is healed, then slowly reintroduce foods that the body wants.

Homework:

1. Offer yourself love. Write on a few pieces of paper, "I love myself" and distribute it throughout your home or work space so you can see it every day. As your eyes glance over the words, you will begin saying it, thinking it and believing it. Self-love is a crucial step we will work on throughout the course of this program. Take that first step and begin saying it to yourself every day, many times a day.
2. Work on raising the vibrations in the home for proper digestion of food/water.

Self-Sabotage
Step Two

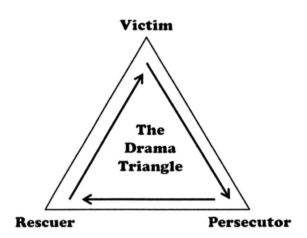

Victim

The Drama Triangle

Rescuer   **Persecutor**

Clear Your Space

Test your client to see if these steps need to be completed before continuing. These steps are found in the Appendix. Always begin your appointments by checking for "attacks."

1. Begin by clearing the space and removing all dark influences/rebellious spirits
2. Remove Self-Destructive Tools of Dark Influences
3. Remove Mind Subconscious suggestions
4. Remove Intimidation Energy
5. Ask for shields of protection

~~~~~~

The Drama Triangle

Step Two is dedicated to education of the drama cycle and self-care. To change a thought pattern we must first see how it plays out in our lives and be capable of seeing the faulty logic. **Our thoughts generate the results in our lives, so to change our lives, we first change our thoughts.** How is this, you say? Well, the process in which we think is a result of our mental state and natural responses to events. This thought process often begins with a stressful event, which produces a thought, which generates an emotion, which can lead to an unhealthy reaction. This reaction typically lacks rational behavior! These responses to the original event are related to your core beliefs about yourself. This cycle is called the **'Drama Triangle'** which is **problem focused**. This cycle consists of 3 roles we tend to play out. We choose to play the victim, the rescuer or the persecutor. We see others as the opposite role in conflict; for instance if you are the victim then the other person is the persecutor while you may be seeking a rescuer. (*In the case of domestic violence, the dynamic is completely different and must not be placed within the confinement of these expectations.*)

The Victim tends to constantly feel as though everyone else is creating the problems they are experiencing in life. The victim sees that the solution rests only in everyone else's power, as others are the creators of the conflict. They will point out the problem and then expect others to fix it while taking no responsibility themselves. The victim believes that if everyone else stops _____ then their problems will cease. In a relationship this will constantly feel like the spouse is the perpetrator, constantly making the victim feel bad or picking on the victim. The victim has no control over their own experiences in life and is living the results of everyone else's choices. The victim will always feel victimized and powerless as they continue to focus on the problem(s).

The Rescuer can be anything we make it to be. It can be in the form of calling up a friend to complain to or seeking out a member of the opposite gender for validation. The rescuer can also be and in the form of an object, such as a tub of ice cream or a cigarette. Music, seclusion, exercise, sleep or whatever it may be to escape the reality of the situation, is all done in an attempt to find a rescuer. When we seek a rescuer we are looking for someone or something to comfort that part that has been wounded and reaffirm our self-worth, typically by blaming the other person. This pattern takes place in many forms within relationships and can lead to divorce as the solution seems impossible to reach. Most times we place a wall or barrier around our hearts to keep others out as a form of self-protection, while missing true connections. However you seek a rescuer, this is an unhealthy dynamic and most are unable to view the true Savior waiting to assist in the healing journey.

The Persecutor can take the form of a person, an event, a culture, an assignment or a trial. This is a way to detach and place the blame upon everyone or everything else. Viewing others as the persecutor is a natural reaction, but ironic enough the persecutor also feels victimized, thus completing the triangle. **Taking responsibility for your own role and discontinuing placing blame on others is the single most difficult step in breaking the cycle of self-sabotage**. Most people are painfully aware of their shortcomings and do not need to be reminded. Remember we are our own worst critics and, therefore, we tend to cover up our guilt by blaming the other person which leads to further pain and heartache for those we love. However, if we choose to live a Christ-like centered life, changing this thought process is an integral step.

The drama triangle is a touchy subject. You may be thinking to yourself, "It's not my fault that he cheated, why should I take the blame" or "I'm not the one with the problem, it's him" or "If only he would show remorse then at least I know he has a conscience" or "He needs to learn, if I don't teach him what he did wrong, then he will never learn." This is exactly the thought process that creates the drama triangle. This drama triangle is a cycle that builds a spiral deeper and deeper into self-sabotage. To break this cycle we must first recognize our roles and who we tend to play in our relationships with others and ourselves. Then choose to break free of this unhealthy pattern. The goal here is to focus upon a better life and better results, and then we will align our current reality with those goals. Learning about the drama triangle is just another step closer towards a better lifestyle.

Conflict Lenses and Lenses of Kindness

When a conflict lens is formed between two individuals, the lens will highlight the flaws or perceived flaws and make obscure the positive qualities in the other person. There can be multiple conflict lenses between individuals. With a sincere intention all of the conflict lenses can be removed and replaced with lenses of kindness. When viewing others through a lens of kindness, the good qualities in others will be highlighted, while the undesirable qualities will be viewed with clarity and understanding.

Conflict lenses are similar to looking through a pair of red goggles where everything you see is tainted red. If you try to see something blue... all you can see is green. You cannot see good or happiness no matter how hard you look. Taking off these old goggles and choosing a new set of lenses is a big process not to be mistaken as simple and mundane. Sometimes these goggles are corded to an event. Sometimes they are being held onto intentionally due to self-disgust and punishment – punishing others or themselves. So these lenses are not a onetime release and done. Free will takes hold in many ways that are positive, but in many ways that are detrimental to the eternal progression. Lingering upon these facts bring no peace to the heart. Even the hardest of hearts feels the love of Christ penetrate deeply in their soul. Many times one may reject God; in this case they are not ready to remove these conflict lenses. It is always a choice. Do not do this without the intention of the client's desire to move forward and experiencing life differently. Many times these lenses are alive and will intensify over time. Innocent they are not; however, since it may be alive, this must be handled quite differently as they will move away and back into place quite rapidly. Catching them is near impossible and however you choose to move forward, they will remain until the energy itself is denied power. Living/lifestyle energies are filled with these lenses. When deep in conflict, these lenses will cloud the perception of reality as emotions take hold. The ability to respond appropriately will feel miserable and impossible; however, Lucifer desires to keep his followers miserable. All are children of God and He loves every single one equally. Love is a powerful healer and many can change their course in life simply with this loving effect.

Finally, these lenses are possibly a rebellious spirit morphing his form into this lens. So test to find out exactly what influence is upon these lenses. At times this may be a good step at the completion of each energy release. Others will be ready to release all at once. You may also find that some conflict lenses will continue to appear until the energy associated with them is released.

1. I bring all conflict lenses to light.
2. I collect all the conflict lenses and separate them into three piles.
    a. One pile is the conflict lenses that I created.
    b. Another pile is the conflict lenses that others created.
    c. And the last is the conflict lenses that were created by rebellious spirits.
3. In the name of Jesus Christ I command all conflict lenses originally created by rebellious spirits to be sent into the portal along with the attached rebellious spirits. I seal the portal never to be reopened.
4. I send light and love into all the remaining conflict lenses.
5. I gather all these lenses together that others have created and I offer forgiveness for those who have created these conflict lenses against me. I choose to see the good in other people regardless of the conflict. I also choose freedom from the negativity that plagues me. Therefore, I choose to love to my enemy and those who despitefully use me, because everyone deserves happiness. However, I may need to create boundaries in order to keep myself safe. Sometimes these lenses are created between families and in that case, I choose to convert these lenses into lenses of kindness.
6. I gather together the conflict lenses that I have created and I choose to see these lenses in their true light along with the event that created the lenses in the first place. I know I am imperfect and progression is slow and sometimes difficult. I offer myself compassion, patience and tolerance. I am safe and I choose to surround myself with love and peace. I choose to see the world through different lenses. I am done seeing the worst in others and myself. I am ready to see the good in the world.
7. I reject all remaining conflict lenses as they no longer serve me.
8. I choose to convert these lenses into lenses of kindness.
    a. I ask for God to convert these into a permanent lens of kindness for the ways in which I view myself and others. I ask that the lens magnify my good qualities and the qualities I see in others. I ask this lens to provide clarity and understanding to undesirable qualities.
        i. Place these between anyone you love or desire to improve the relationship
        ii. This works fantastic in a marriage if you are working on a couple!

~~~~~~

Self-Talk

Your external world is a reflection of your internal world. Quite simply self-talk is the story you play out in your head and what you tell yourself, but is spoken as fact when it is actually just an opinion. For example, you look in the mirror at yourself and think, "I am so fat, how could anybody love me when I look like this?" or "If I had a different result then I'd change and be happy" or in a heated discussion with a loved one if they offend or hurt your feelings, you may think to yourself, "I am a failure and keep screwing everything up." This self-talk reflects your emotions and perception of the events taking place. You are your own worst critic; self-talk is the manner in which we sabotage the ability to think clearly and rationally especially within conflict. Breaking this cycle is a critical step that begins with awareness and accountability.

Awareness of where negative self-talk originated may surprise you. Once it becomes habit, you'll see it's been a part of your life subconsciously. However, you can probably recognize when the Holy Ghost touches your heart, but can you decipher when the adversary is deceiving you? Most negative self-talk is influenced by the rebellion, but becomes a natural thought pattern through self-loathing.

Self-talk gains power through emotions. When you are emotionally connected to a memory, that emotional memory will create neural pathways in the brain. These new patterns will become your new comfort zone. Therefore, if life's trials create faulty core beliefs, the emotional memory can be reflected upon and still contain the emotional attachment just as powerful as the day it was created. Let's test this theory. I want you to remember the last argument you had with a spouse or friend. Think about what happened and what was said. Are you becoming emotional: upset, angry, feeling as though the argument is still occurring? This is due to the hormonal reaction to the emotions. With energy work, we work on changing this intense energy from the past and the hormonal reaction while forming a new thought pattern. Your self-talk holds the same power. When you look in the mirror, do you see yourself as "needing improvement?" Do you only focus on the areas of your body you do not like? What thoughts run through your head as you peer at your own reflection? This self-talk can be life affirming or life draining. It is all within you. The solution is within your own mind and part of the work we will be doing in this program.

When we are shifting this dynamic, it is just as critical to become emotionally attached to the new empowering thought process. When your memory focuses upon an event the emotions solidify the memory. For instance, in school you may have memorized information to pass a test. Is this information still accessible to you 10 years later? What if you learned about the pioneers through an experience where you watched an emotional video or visited a pioneer home? When you become emotionally attached to a story, you remember details. Our goals are to create such powerful self-talk that when you look in the mirror, you feel incredible gratitude for your body and you feel a deep sense of love and respect for yourself. Not simply just memorized words without an emotional attachment.

~~~~~~

Faulty Core Beliefs / Limiting Beliefs

A faulty core belief is typically created due to past experiences or a misinterpretation of behavior. If a dating experience in life created a belief such as: "All men are cheaters" or "All women are drama queens," this is obviously not fact. However, if this is your core belief, you'll believe it as a fact, thus changing the way you see the opposite gender. A **Limiting Belief** typically is an "I can't because" statement which is the verbal thought process. A limiting belief is a derivative of a faulty core belief. While affirmations lead to empowering core beliefs. For example; if your core belief is "All men are cheaters," then your limiting belief is "I can't trust men; I will never allow another man into my life." Or "I'm not good enough; otherwise, he wouldn't have wanted another woman." Most core beliefs are simple and straightforward while the limiting belief is emotional and there may be hundreds of limiting beliefs stemming from one faulty core belief. Most core and limiting beliefs expose themselves as self-talk. You can easily find your own thought patterns by listening to your self-talk.

Our comfort zones are places we have built, but does your comfort zone bring you happiness? Most likely everything you want is outside this comfort zone. Your thought patterns are comfort zones. Changing these thoughts may make you feel uncomfortable at first as you are stepping out of your comfort zone. Change takes effort, humility and dedication, but contains growth opportunities. Our past is an opportunity to grow, learn and heal; changing your perspective is the path towards healing. Awareness assists you in knowing what change needs to occur. Your faulty core beliefs are creating the circumstances you are currently living. These beliefs drive your life and how you respond to triggers.

Limiting beliefs are created from an unconscious reaction. A limiting belief is a lie we tell ourselves that will end up sabotaging any progress we pursue. Anything you say to yourself to justify why it isn't working out for you is a limiting belief. This can also be seen as an automatic thought response that becomes a pattern of thinking. Limiting beliefs are created by our perception of the world based upon our misunderstanding of the event. An example of this is, if the core belief is "I can't succeed;" then the unconscious reaction to a new experience would be "What's the point in trying anyway, it's not like I can afford it and nobody ever helps me. Nobody cares about me and the whole world is against me." The end result would be giving up on a dream or quitting, therefore leading towards solidifying the victimhood belief and lifestyle.

The first thing to do is, acknowledge that these are beliefs, NOT truths! **"When we argue for our limitations, we get to keep them**." – Evelyn Waugh. Here's the place where choice comes in. Which are you more interested in: defending your limitations or achieving your goals? You choose. There's an important detail here. When you realize you desire a change, it can feel intimidating, because your current life traps you in the path you previously set. Change takes effort and stepping out of your comfort zone means changing your lifestyle. The people in your life will be affected by your transformation. Your home, your job, everything is your creation and when you desire change, resistance is guaranteed. So baby steps and small changes over time is the true path towards a total transformation. Remember to feed yourself love and over time the rest will fall into place. As we release the negativity from the past, this change will become easier and easier. Remember you are not alone!

Let's try on a different belief – a belief that is aligned with what you want or your vision for your future that you are passionately pursuing. Let's dismantle and reword the above limiting beliefs to take on a positive perspective or twist. If we take our example phrase and apply an empowering core belief of "I am worthy," your conscious thought would be "I am excited to try something new regardless of whether I succeed or not, the growth process will bring about opportunities and I take responsibility for my own needs. I am lucky to have such a wonderful support system in place." Therefore, coming from and leading to a Conscious Creator Mindset.

What are your current limiting beliefs or faulty core beliefs? (brainstorm and/or muscle test with the chart in the Appendix on page 132):

_____

_____

_____

_____

_____

_____

What is your self-talk? What phrases do you say to yourself when you look in the mirror? What do you think about yourself when something "bad" happens? What life draining things do you say to yourself?

_____

_____

_____

_____

When things go right in life, when you are having a really good day and you feel good about yourself; what life affirming things do you say to yourself?

_____

_____

_____

_____

~~~~~~

Assignments

Energy Work:

1. Release the victim dark energy or the revenge/death dark energies or the addiction dark or the dark dark energy.
2. Test for organ function and monitor the progress through the 12 steps.
3. Be aware that foods tested prior will fluctuate based on the release of energies and the healing of the organs.
4. Work on toxins and infections. (These steps are found in the Spirit Code program)

Homework: Focus on your self-talk and be aware of the words you feed yourself on a daily basis. Where did these thoughts originate? Was it someone else's words or your own? Are your expectations too high or can you meet them? Is your self-talk life affirming or life draining? Take notes and discuss with your energy healer.

Self-Sabotage
Step Three

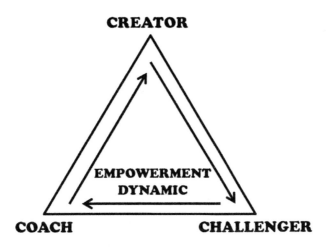

CREATOR

EMPOWERMENT DYNAMIC

COACH   **CHALLENGER**

Clear Your Space

Test your client to see if these steps need to be completed before continuing. These steps are found in the Appendix. Always begin your appointments by checking for "attacks."

1. Begin by clearing the space and removing all dark influences/rebellious spirits
2. Remove Self-Destructive Tools of Dark Influences
3. Remove Mind Subconscious suggestions
4. Remove Intimidation Energy
5. Ask for shields of protection

~~~~~~

The Empowerment Dynamic

When you are ready to shift your perspective from the Drama Triangle, we step into the **Empowerment Dynamic** which is **solution focused**. You can play a part as the Creator, the Coach or the Challenger. In this dynamic we choose a role and see others in the opposite roles.

With the Empowerment Dynamic you can choose to step into your life as a creator, shedding the victimhood of the drama triangle. As a creator you focus upon the desired outcome, and then manifest this outcome, thus producing satisfying results. **A creator is vision focused**

and passion motivated. When you become passionate about your vision for your life, you naturally desire to align your actions with what you want to manifest. A creator is filled with power, power to create. This power is shared with others as we begin to see others in their own right. A creator is actually a **co-creator with God** and thus collaborating in accordance with God's will. A creator is humble and patient with the process. The creator sees others in life as a coach or a challenger, because they view life as a growing opportunity. A creator doesn't fight the experiences or fall victim to them, a creator will choose to enjoy the ride and allow the experiences to offer growth and perspective.

The Creator: will take the place of the victim. The creator sees every experience in life as an opportunity for growth. The creator has the power to create anything they desire simply by believing it is possible and taking the steps to align their daily choices with that ultimate goal. The creator is aware of their self-talk and their core beliefs and chooses to see the best in themselves and others. When life throws a curveball or they face opposition, the creator will look at the event differently as others cannot shake their self-worth. They will see events as a challenge or an opportunity for growth. For example, I was attending a seminar for personal development and my life coach was the presenter. A friend of mine was triggered and angrily speaking against the coach; so I sat down with my coach who I highly admire and told him what was being said. His response spoke volumes to me. He said, "It doesn't hurt because I know it's not true, that is not the story I have for myself." I sat and pondered his words as I realized how difficult it is to receive criticism. He was able to respond consciously and with Christ-like love for his accusers because he knew within himself the truth. I believe this is the deeper meaning behind being a creator. A creator is conscious or mindful of the present while having empowering core beliefs to back up the automatic emotional response so the reaction is empowering. The creator no longer feels victimized, they instead feel empowered which leads to an uplifting energy radiating from your being that others can feel.

The Coach: helps the creator evaluate and use their power. Much like a coach for a sporting event, they support you and hold you accountable while pushing you outside of your comfort zone. A coach may also encourage you to set healthy boundaries. They will provoke thought and encourage you to think outside the box by asking you questions to solve a problem. They will help you to reach your ultimate purpose in life by encouraging you to move forward when life becomes challenging. When you are in the role of the creator, a coach will be a spouse, a friend or a leader and will take the place of the rescuer.

The Challenger: encourages learning and growth opportunities. A challenger could be a person in your life or a difficult project at work or an event that presents distress. A challenger takes the place of the persecutor. When we stand in our power as creators, the other roles fall into place. This is when we face trials as a challenge to overcome and we can offer love to ourselves or patience to accomplish the task at a steady pace. When we are ready to face the trials with a new understanding and love for all mankind, we shift even higher into a more Christ-like dynamic. Simply by shifting the perspective in life and seeing the world as a gift for progression from a loving Father in Heaven, we will open a world of understanding and love for others even when they may pose trials in life.

I would like to offer a plan to assist you in switching your perspective and choosing another role in your life and in your relationships. We will also shift your core belief system about yourself which produces these natural emotion responses. Let's agree that the way you have been <u>reacting</u> in your life has not worked… Instead, let's become consciously mindful of words, thoughts and actions.

~~~~~~

Grounding with the Earth

Energy work: When we are "grounded" we have the ability to draw strength from the earth. The earth can share healing energy and spiritual nutrients with our spirits and bodies. Consider the compound charts, many of those energies are offered to us by the earth. The earth has an incredible desire for us to be healthy and wants to support us in our healing efforts. Since the earth is holy and respects our agency, she waits until we call upon her for help. Our Father in heaven and Savior created this earth for the purpose of sustaining all we need for life. As we look to our Father and Savior for help we can also turn towards the earth for assistance. Keep in mind, the spirits of the earth, sun and other heavenly bodies are all connected to the network of angels. This network is one with God and they each desire to help us in their own special way. As you may have already noticed, some of our energy releases utilized tools and energy offered to us by heavenly bodies, such as the Sun, Pluto, and Jupiter.

Grounding is particularly important for when the earth makes dramatic shifts energetically and physically as we approach the second coming of our Savior. The grounding will help balance our spirits and help us to "go with the flow." Picture the root of a giant redwood tree. Imagine how deep and sturdy these roots are. The roots provide support to the tree and absorb nutrients from the earth. We will form energetic roots that are similar to the roots of a giant tree.

Visualization: Close your eyes and imagine yourself standing outside in the soil with bare feet. The sun is upon your back and the smell of the air is fresh like a forest. Stand very still and see roots growing out of your feet and into the earth. They will start off as small shoots and spread out deeper and deeper into the earth. Invite the earth to continually offer you her energy and support in any manner that she deems beneficial to you through these roots. Trust in her abilities to do this, since she has done this for many generations. Continue expanding your roots while forming a respect for the earth's life giving soils. You can keep growing your roots as deep as you'd like, creating a solid root system. Also, invite in the healing beneficial elements of the sun at your head to strengthen your body, mind, and spirit as you act as an energy conductor between the earth and the sun. Soak up the healing energy being offered in this visualization.

~~~~~~

Find Your Destination

This life you are currently living is your creation; the people in your life, your home, job, finances, love, family, etc. You are the creator of this life you are currently living, which means you have the same power to change anything that is not in alignment with your goals. When you shift your focus from being a victim of your life to being the creator of your life, what changes might you notice? How does this empower you to create change? Is this a perspective you would like to create in your own life? What would your life look like if you stepped into the role of a creator?

Visualization #1: What you can imagine, you can create. Your mind believes what it can envision; therefore, the story that you see, your mind will have power to create change. So please, close your eyes. Imagine yourself lounging in a safe space, your home, the beach, the mountains, or anywhere else you feel peaceful and content. This needs to be a place of solitude where you are free to experience your dreams. Look around at your current location; breathe deeply and slowly. Across the sky is a video of your life. Your childhood begins to play showing all the trials and triumphs. As you watch, offer yourself compassion and understanding. See how these events have taught and changed you. As the scene speeds up into your youth, you can see the full picture of events playing out that created your interpretation of the world. Allow forgiveness to overwhelm your heart as you view these events. Remind yourself that you are a lovable and better person for these experiences. Now, the scene speeds up to your young adult life. You choose the path for your life and go out on your own. Take a deep breath as you allow your heart to fill with love and gratitude for all the challenges which taught you how to care for yourself. Now the scene speeds up to this moment in your life; however, as you look around you can fully comprehend how everything you are experiencing is a creation of your choices and your past. Invite Christ to view this scene with you, see him standing to your side. Ask Him to assist you (as you are His co-creator) to create a new understanding and perspective shift, to allow an alignment with your higher self. He says to you, "This is your life, live it well." All at once you realize this is your only chance to experience life, your only chance to be you, to live your dreams, and to create your ideal life. He reminds you, "You are loved. You are a royal child of God of infinite worth, there is nobody in the world exactly like you, you are My creation, you are perfect in the sight of the God, and you are perfect exactly as you are right now." Allow these encouraging words to flow through you and focus upon a life filled with your wildest dreams; everything you could ever want for yourself or others. Focus on living the life that you desire most. Think of the changes that must take place first, in order to experience this change. Now look at the film and as it speeds up one year in the future, see how these changes are taking place to create new results in your life. These changes are naturally taking place as you are aligning with that ultimate vision for your life.

1. What needs to take place first in order to experience your dreams?
2. What does this version of your life look like?

As you are watching this video of your life you are experiencing joy and happiness like you've never experienced before. Give yourself permission to experience happiness. Recognize the effort that has taken place to create the results you desire. Watch as you work towards your goal with passion, which is motivating you to work harder and serve more. Five years speed by in the video of living your dreams, living in a space of pure happiness where you enjoy every moment of your life. Your thoughts naturally take you to a place of self-love and living in a

Christ-like manner, because you have created this version of your life – a life centered around living your purpose and your dream. You have invited God into every avenue of your existence. Your relationship with Him is the solid stable ground you stand upon, every footstep leads you along the path He is guiding. Your effort has created your desired results and you are living the life of your dreams. Take a moment to look around this life you are living five years in the future.

1. Is this reality worth the effort it took to create?
2. How has this direction changed your life, family and your future opportunities?

Once again the video speeds up another five years. Your life vision has snowballed into so much more than you could have ever imagined possible. These years have reshaped your version of reality and your understanding of the world. Your new empowering core beliefs have become a way of life, created out of your experiences. You see the world as opportunity, you lead others towards their goals, you have not only arrived at your dreams, but you have solidified them and have become a completely different person. You are so overfilled with gratitude that you took a huge step in your life, which shifted events to lead you to the person you've become today. This places you 10 full years into your future; you are a whole new person and with Christ standing at your side, you look at His eyes and see they are welling up with tears of joy. You embrace and thank Him for offering you this gift of life to experience, grow and learn to become more like Him.

1. What does your life look like 10 years in the future?
2. Are you ready to align your current life with this vision of the future?

Once again, within this safe space and your heart filled with emotions, we are going to watch these last 10 years rewind back to the present day – your present life, your current reality, and your current thoughts. Offer Christ gratitude for showing you a better way to live your life. Open your eyes, I want you to experience what is going through your mind and allow the emotions to flow. I want you to focus upon this truth – this is YOUR life, this is your one chance to live and experience life.

1. Where has your life been heading on your current path vs. where do you prefer your life to take you?
2. What changes are necessary to align your life with your life's vision?
3. What's stopping you from aligning your life with this reality?

~~~~~~

Search and Rescue

Visualization #2: Let's take another journey together today. Close your eyes again and I want you to imagine someone knocking on the front door. You walk to the door and open it up to find Jesus Christ standing before you. He beckons for you to come with Him. He says to you, "It is time." He takes your hand and leads you into a cloud that is mysteriously in front of your home, it is welcoming and filled with light and love. As you walk in this cloud with Christ holding your hand, you realize you are now in the midst of the worst moment of your past. The one moment that holds you hostage in your memories as you struggle to move past this event you endured. You see yourself in this horrible moment and you feel so many emotions. Your breath catches in your throat and you turn to Christ, frightened and needing His help. He says, "Go comfort yourself. Tell yourself it will all be okay." So you walk over to the younger version of you and you embrace. You proceed to say everything to your younger self that you needed to hear in that moment; words of counsel, comfort, and kindness. (Pause a moment)

Now take the hand of your younger self and invite them to come with you outside. As you step outside, another person approaches from the cloud and as they come closer you recognize them. It's you, but it's the celestialized version of you coming to comfort both of you. This higher version embraces the both of you and offers counsel and guidance and tells you everything you need to hear right now. (*Pause a moment*) Christ joins you and reminds you, "You have never been alone; these trials have been for your good. You are a better person for all your experiences this life has brought. Forgive those who have wronged you. Forgive yourself for wronging others. Come unto me for healing; you are loved so dearly. Your potential is great. Love yourself as I love you." At the conclusion of the Savior's words, the higher version of you smiles and walks back into the cloud. You turn to the younger version of you and embrace once again. Offer yourself compassion for the events they are currently experiencing. The younger version of you says, "You are safe now. Thank you for coming back for me, I will be ok… I see now that I am a glorious child of God and I can overcome all because of the love of my Savior. Go and live the life we have always dreamed of." So you turn and walk back into the cloud, as Christ remains in the past with your younger self. Come back into your home and offer gratitude for the opportunity to come to peace with your experiences. Say a prayer in this moment and speak to your Father in Heaven about what just transpired.

(*Pause a moment*)

Umbilical Cord

We have Heavenly Parents; a Father and a Mother. A mother's job is to love, protect, and nurture. A father's job is to lead, guide and teach. There is a powerful cord we have with our Heavenly Mother. It is much like an umbilical cord where She offers us constant love and nourishment. However, throughout our lives this connection can become knotted due to painful experiences as we block out Her love **sub**consciously. This connection is holy and cannot be touched by us. Mother will not remove the knots without our consent either. You can test how many knots are in your "umbilical cord" with Heavenly Mother. Close your eyes and say a private prayer, if you so choose, and ask Heavenly Mother to remove these knots so you may be able to more fully experience the love She has to offer you throughout your life.

This is done privately and humbly as this relationship is sacred.

Extra Sensory Perception

Extra Sensory Perception (ESP) also known as the 6th sense: This is a sense that allows communication with God. We are all born with this functioning at 100%. Imagine this sense as a spot in the front of the head, with a direct cord – a bright, sacred, holy cord to our Father in heaven. A block has been created within this connection. This block has been created by you and interferes with the communication offered through the connection. This sense is the FIRST sense to become blocked to the point where it doesn't even exist or at least it isn't even recognized as a natural gift from God for all mankind. This sense will die due to rejection, a lack of acceptance in the world or too many unclean spirits attacking this sense. This sense is one of the most basic and critical to protect. God sent us here without our memories, but He allowed this communication. It was never meant to die or burn out or become blocked, this is strictly one of Lucifer's ploys to draw us away from God.

1. Test to see what percentage of the ESP is open:_____
2. Test to see what percentage of the ESP blocked/rejected:_____
3. Test to see what percentage of the ESP burnt out/dead:_____

There are two types of blocks: **protection** and **rejection**. The protection block is placed onto this sense by our spirit, because our spirit wants this divine connection to be protected. The rejection block has been placed onto the sense, because we have chosen to reject the communication offered by God. To remove the blocks, there are 3 steps that must be taken. The second and third steps for the protection block are essentially the same as the second and third steps for the rejection block, so they can be done together. The steps are quite personal and beyond repetition. It must be sincere and felt to be true in the spirit; you cannot lie to your spirit.

Protection Block:

1. The **first** stage is to atone by coming to peace with your spirit regarding the sinful actions of the past. Accepting the atonement for this step must be so personal that the spirit itself feels safe. Remember "safe" references protecting the relationship with God as the spirit naturally recognizes the intense sacredness of this connection.

2. The **second** step is asking God. Communicate your intentions with our Father and involve Him in this, as it is a SHARED connection with the most sacred being. The extra sensory perception is too holy to touch, just like the umbilical cord. (*Note: this does not include the block.*)

3. So step **three** is to convert the block into a sliver of wood for the cross and offer it to the Lord.

Rejection Block: When the block is due to rejection, the process is similar with three steps but in the atonement step, this is **directed to the rejection of God's affection**.

Symbology of the Cross: Related scripture (King James Version)

Mark 8: 34

34 And when he had called the people *unto him* with his disciples also, he said unto them, Whosoever will come after me, let him deny himself, and **take up his cross**, and follow me.

Chakra Direction: The spinning of the crown chakra. To receive the maximum benefits of this sense, let's shift the chakra flow. They all face forward, but the crown chakra can flip and rotate upwards towards God. When the light from the chakra faces forward it blocks out the light and communication flow, but when facing upwards, the flow is opened up. Also the rotation of these chakras are intertwined with the flow from God and the ESP sense. When these three twist together and magnify their connection, the reception increases.

When you release the block there's still more to receive the proper function of the ESP. We need to communicate with the switches and electrical wiring of the brain and of course remind the body of its proper functioning. This can be done by stating, "I awaken the Fibonacci sequence within my mind and spirit and invite the flow of the golden ratio to flow through my being." You also need to change your mindset. If you still believe that you cannot see angels, then you cannot. You must change your approach at life and the spirit world. Changing your belief is the only way to work with this sense and it is the only way to keep it alive and healthy and clean.

Dead Sense: Correction goes beyond reminding the sense of its creation. Remember this is holy and connected to God; therefore, the offering is not removed. The sense is strictly deadened within you. The spirit never dies, but the body does. When the body passes away and begins to deteriorate, the spirit is partially affected as the connection with the body is so powerful; the gratitude for the body, the remorse, the intense bond does not die even after the body decomposes. But our Father through the atonement offers hope for reuniting the body and the spirit. Let's simplify how this relates to the ESP; this perception is connected in a sacred bond to God and your spirit. God never passes away, neither does the spirit, but the body that houses the spirit does. This ESP is a part of the spirit AND the mind. God's attachment to you does not cease due to the death of this perception. Our limited mind breaks down the full meaning of this perception; it is beyond your full capacity to grasp during this mortal probation. In other words, you must go forward with faith and trust our Father in Heaven. So regarding the death of this sense – the resurrection offers us hope, but it does not occur during our perception of time. It is beyond our ability as the resurrection is Godly. This, we cannot stress enough, it is as if your umbilical cord to Mother had dried up and rotted off. She is still connected, but the direct flow is gone… There is hope, there is always hope, but it is best to take the necessary steps to create other bonds with our Father, until your righteousness is rewarded with a new extra sensory perception… this means it will have to be created by God. You may ask God to create a new one, since His love for you remains. If it is not done immediately, this is not meant to punish, it is to help assist you to fully atone. A deadened ESP doesn't happen by chance. Everyone has a story and each story is special in its own respect, we will not be able to explain the reasons behind our Father's decision, as each is special and complicated.

Assignments

Energy work:

1. Release another energy based on the needs of the client. If they test positive for the Victim Dark energy be sure to release this now.
2. Invite and absorb into the meridian the pure Love of God continuously for _____ days and to be distributed throughout the body, mind and spirit. Add any additional healthy emotions from the chart in the Appendix on page 127.
3. Create a compound as needed for healing.
4. Continue working on toxins and infections. (These steps are found in the Spirit Code program)

Homework Affirmations: Say these every day, _____ times a day to create new thought patterns. This will take conscious daily effort to retrain the mind.

1. _____
2. _____
3. _____
4. _____
5. _____

Self-Sabotage
Step Four

Clear Your Space

Test your client to see if these steps need to be completed before continuing. These steps are found in the Appendix. Always begin your appointments by checking for "attacks."

1. Begin by clearing the space and removing all dark influences/rebellious spirits
2. Remove Self-Destructive Tools of Dark Influences
3. Remove Mind Subconscious suggestions
4. Remove Intimidation Energy
5. Ask for shields of protection

~~~~~~

Your Perfectly Designed Body

God created your body and your spirit. Your body is the temple for your spirit which means your spirit is far more sacred than you may have realized. Your body is an amazing creation built perfectly to heal itself. Think of the last time you got a cut on your arm; did this cut get infected or continue getting worse and crack open your arm until the whole arm fell off? Of course not. That's not how the body is created. Most likely your arm naturally clotted the blood, naturally formed a scab and naturally healed the skin to look perfectly new over time. Maybe the cut was deeper, but essentially, the body healed the injury through no real effort on your part. Why is this? Your body is ALIVE! Every cell is alive and moving, because you are complete ENERGY! You exist due to the energy of your body.

God made your existence possible: your lungs breathe, your heart beats, your body moves according to your will and you can think/act/speak for yourself. Since your body was created by God, anything unholy or not created by God will present physical symptoms. Your symptoms are a way for your body to communicate with you that something is wrong and needs to change. For instance: God created love, forgiveness, compassion, humility, patience, etc. However, Lucifer created anger, hate, spite, revenge, self-loathing, criticism, judgment, etc. So when you experience these negative emotions or energies, your body sees them as foreign and toxic. Your body may store these toxic energies by creating more fat cells for protecting you from the toxicity within. Your body may place the energy within your muscles presenting symptoms of fibromyalgia or back spasms. Your body may store this energy in your lungs showing symptoms of anxiety or asthma. Your body could even store the negative energy as excess dense tissue which is cancer. Your emotions create a hormonal reaction and excess toxins due to these emotions which also creates physical symptoms.

Once we can change our thought patterns, we can heal/release the past negative energies and assist the body in the healing process. An effective way to change our lifestyle is through personal development work, combined with energy work and tapping. This creates a dynamic opportunity to heal in the spirit, mind and body.

~~~~~~

Manager and Boxes/Balls

When we experience an intense dark energy, we give away our power to a rebellious spirit that acts as a "manager." He then manages the compartments in our minds. The compartments: men have boxes and women have balls they are juggling. We found that ideally men have 24 boxes and women have 24 balls. Some categories include: food, sleep, entertainment, work, family, etc. Many people have far too many boxes/balls; we have also found some people have far too little balls/boxes. Once a manager is given power, you'll find either missing balls/boxes or an excess. Test yourself and your client for how many balls/boxes you have in your mind.

When we experience a devastating trial and our thoughts lead us away from God, we invite rebellious spirits into our presence (typically subconsciously). A rebellious spirit that is contracted as a manager will create an excess of clutter in the mind, causing an overwhelming amount of tasks or responsibilities where you may struggle to focus on a task. Rebellious spirits can be found within a person's mind or body as they do not respect agency. Most everyone has a manager influencing the boxes/balls within their mind as they have given away their power to someone else to take the responsibility. Think of the last time you expected someone else to fix your symptoms with a pill or the last time you blamed someone else when things went wrong. We have given away our power little by little and stopped taking responsibility for ourselves, because we are imperfect and accepting these imperfections is very difficult. It's easier to blame others or expect others to fix us.

The manager is there because of an energy that opened the door to the mind. These managers can be very tricky to remove. This energy was formed due to your emotional and thought reaction to an event. This dark energy needs to be removed first. (Removal of the dark energy is a very detailed process and must be done properly as found in the Spirit Code program). This will remove a lot of the power that the manager has, making it much easier to proceed. However, there is also a portal, so let's do this the fast way and remove them both at the same time.

Ask your client: Do you want a rebellious spirit influencing your thoughts? Would you want to hear the Holy Ghost more clearly? Test if there is a manager and a portal. Test to see what type of portal: wormhole, fear, time, electrical or a basic portal. Test to see how many boxes/balls there are in the mind.

Energy Work:

1. Bring to light all negative energy, managers, portals, rebellious spirits and cords.
2. Identify (muscle test the options below) what type of portal is connected to the manager and then follow the steps. There are many types of portals; however, the most commonly used portals are listed below. We have found that the managers prefer to form a wormhole.

   a. **Wormhole:** It is open in the past, present and future.
      i. Fold the wormhole in half so that the past is lying on top of the future.
      ii. Take the openings in the past and the future and interlace them together.
      iii. Command all the energy in the spirit, mind and body that is connected to this manager to be thrown into the present opening as if the portal was a giant magnet sucking all the energy into the portal.
      iv. Command all excess boxes/balls that were not self-created to also be thrown into the present opening (pause a few moments).
      v. Ask for the assistance of silver to zip up the present opening of the portal.
      vi. Remove the cords: Detach / Cut with the Sword of the Rebellion / Release / Remove

   b. **General Portal:**
      i. Command all the energy in the spirit, mind and body that is connected to this manager to be thrown into the portal as if the portal was a giant magnet sucking all the energy into the portal.
      ii. Command all excess boxes/balls that were not self-created to also be thrown into the portal (pause a few moments).
      iii. In the name of Jesus Christ command that the portal be sealed.
      iv. Remove the cords: Detach / Cut with the Sword of the Rebellion / Release / Remove

   c. **Electrical Portals:** These are portal with electricity flowing through them. This allows the portals to be connected to electrical devices.
      i. Attach one end of a cobalt grounding line to the earth.
      ii. Attach the other end to the cord that is connected to the portal (or that the portal is on). This will drain the electricity and it will then become a general portal that is commonly used.
      iii. Command all the energy in the spirit, mind and body that is connected to this manager to be thrown into the portal.
      iv. Command all excess boxes/balls that were not self-created to also be thrown into the portal (pause a few moments).
      v. In the name of Jesus Christ command that the portal be sealed.
      vi. Remove the cords: Detach / Cut with the Sword of the Rebellion / Release / Remove

   d. **Time portal:** Sealing a time portal must be sealed at a different time points in time. You need to identify the time in which the portal exists, so you can close it in each time period. As an example: The portal may exist in the present, 943 years in the past and 943 years in the future. Seal it in the past, present and future.

      i. First: Command that the rebellious spirits (*this does not include the manager*) be removed and placed into the portals. <u>Command that the spirits be trapped in a time loop within the portals.</u>

      ii. Command all the energy in the spirit, mind and body that is connected to this manager to be thrown into the portal.

      iii. Command all excess boxes/balls that were not self-created to also be thrown into the portal (pause a few moments).

      iv. Ask for the heat of the sun to cauterize each portal – in the past, present and future.

      v. Banish the portals from reality.

      vi. Remove the cords: Detach / Cut with the Fortified Time Sword (or the Sun Sword) / Release / Remove

3. There is a contract involved so command the contract to be placed in your hands and test which method is best for cleansing the contract and then cleanse the names from contract:

    a. Wash the contract with the living waters

    b. Burn the contract

    c. Baptize the contract in the Jordan River

    d. Bathe the contract in tears of forgiveness

4. Step in between the boxes/balls and the manager. This step is very important; this needs to be done with confidence. You are showing that you now have taken back the power within your mind. Say with confidence – "I choose to be the manager of my own mind; it is time for you to leave!"

5. Close your eyes and invite the light of Christ to shine forth from your body and hands and into the remaining boxes. Imagine them compartmentalizing themselves into the proper sequence with the proper number and the sub-compartments into their proper box.

6. For the men, place the magnets into the correct locations based upon the proper sequencing (they are what keeps the boxes in place). For women imagine these balls becoming light as a feather by releasing all negative energy from within each ball.

7. Turn to the manager and ask for a Golden Light Sword. Cut all of the strings/chains between the boxes/balls and the manager. The strings attached to the boxes will dissolve on their own due to the power of the sword.

8. Command the manager to depart: "It is now time for you to leave; your services are no longer desired." Offer some compassion as their life is miserable. Offer an act of kindness. "You have 3 choices: 1) Depart. 2) If you attack; I will cast you out. 3) Repent and become an angel in training."

    a. Wait a few moments to see what they chose, you can test or go based off your emotions. If you feel scared, quickly recognize it is time to cast them out and do so in the name of Jesus Christ with your right arm to the square. If you feel sad; they probably left. If you feel the spirit touch your heart; they have chosen to turn towards God. Remember these are disembodied spirits and they are our brothers and sisters who have lost their way, most likely due to tragedy.

9. Now test to see how many boxes/balls remain. Test to be sure the portal is sealed. Test to be sure the rebellious spirit has departed or become an angel in training.

The importance of this step will become more known to you as you recognize that within conflict situations you'll be more capable of choosing a different path. You'll more effectively be able to change your core beliefs and begin thinking more heavenly. Your shields will remain longer and fewer attacks may occur. Your confidence may boost and you can control your self-talk more.

~~~~~~

Automatic Responses Based off Core Beliefs

Let's discuss how our thought process affects our actions and why it's so critical to learn from the example of Jesus Christ in keeping our thoughts holy. Your core beliefs create an automatic thought process when a trigger occurs which may be your faulty self-talk. This automatic thought process creates an emotional response which is often irrational and untrue, but believed as truth. This response is caused by the automatic thought process, not the event itself. This response then naturally leads to a specific resulting behavior. Let's discuss what this means and why it is vital to understand.

- **Trigger:** Ruth has saved up her money for a particular movie she has been dying to see so she invites her best friend, Jane, to come along. Ruth gets a babysitter, cleans the house, schedules work, pampers herself and gets totally excited for a much needed girls night out. Last minute Jane invites another person to join the girls night, but this person has already seen the movie so Jane calls Ruth to make a last minute change in the movie plans…

- **Faulty core belief:** So when Ruth's faulty core belief is "I'm worthless, nobody cares, I hate myself, I am a victim" Then her automatic thought response will fall into place.

- **Automatic thought response:** "I saved up just for this movie I have been dying to see. I can't afford to go again. Why did she invite someone else and now they are changing the plans. That's not fair. Now I will never see the movie I wanted, obviously my opinion doesn't matter. They would probably even prefer to just go without me. Is she even my friend? Doesn't she care at all about me? I can't afford to go out twice, this isn't fair to me."

- **Automatic emotional response:** feeling hurt, betrayed, rejected, alone, and disrespected.

- **Resulting Behavior:** It is natural to want to feel better so Ruth may stay at home and over eat a carton of ice cream. Or Ruth will call up another friend seeking validation or to complain looking for comfort. Ruth might have an addictive habit such as shopping, eating, smoking, drinking, or sleeping which helps her to feel better. Or Ruth may still go out with her friends, but spit out passive aggressive comments the whole time trying to get them to feel bad for disappointing her. She might even get into a fight with her husband as she takes out her hurt feelings on someone else. Possibly Ruth will even get into a fight with Jane because she wants Jane to know how much she's hurting.

This is the automatic thought responses and automatic emotional responses. This is not something you can easily control if the core belief is faulty. It is not true that Ruth's friend doesn't care, but it is believed as truth due to Jane's actions. So Ruth believes that Jane is the one who needs to change in order for a solution or resolution. This creates the Drama Triangle as you focus on the problem. You can see how quickly the drama triangle can explode into an emotional dilemma, how one can feel victimized, and will blame others for their emotions. In this scenario, Jane has really done no harm, but her actions are misrepresented due to the self-talk Ruth automatically experienced. Jane may feel victimized and so may Ruth as they both see the other as the perpetrator.

Let's rewrite this scenario and see how an empowering core belief may change the situation. Remember the solution is not to control or change the other person or to force them to see things your way. That is not a healthy or successful solution either. Rather we will shift the core beliefs and see how the response changes. Same trigger, same initial story.

- **Empowering core belief:** Let's say Ruth's core belief is: "I am loved, I am lovable, I am special, I matter, I am the creator of my life" then this will be her automatic thought response to the trigger:

- **Automatic thought response:** (rational self-talk) – "I can be flexible regarding the movie, it is more important to have that special time with friends. Inviting other friends doesn't mean I am any less important, in fact it gives me an opportunity to make another friend. Plus, I can always speak up and tell them how important the other movie is to me, maybe she won't mind seeing it again, but I bet any movie we see will be a blast."

- **Automatic emotional response:** Excitement to have a special night out with friends. Gratitude to have friends and the desire to make new friends.

- **Resulting Behavior:** Ruth participates in the girl's night out, all the while feeding herself love and sharing her friendship with others. She may realize what's truly important in life and shine her light to bless others while creating an epic evening. Ruth is filled with joy because she chooses to see the best in others and herself. Everyone is getting along and having a fantastic night out.

Can you see how easily the original mood or core belief can change the whole experience? Nothing changed about Ruth's friends. All that changed was her core belief which led to automatic responses and changed the entire course of events. No man can break an addiction simply by trying to resist the temptation; however when you do personal development work to fix the "cause", the change just comes naturally. Most patterns or habits take a long time to correct. It takes 90 days to form a new habit.

Let's discuss times in your life where either of these thought processes were prevalent. Can you give me some examples of your own life where you were triggered? Can you recognize where these original thoughts occurred? (Possibly homework, important to recognize these within your own life)

Trigger:_____

_____

Automatic Thought Response: _____

_____

Automatic Emotional Response:_____

_____

Resulting Behavior:_____

_____

Trigger:_____

_____

Automatic Thought Response: _____

_____

Automatic Emotional Response:_____

_____

Resulting Behavior:_____

_____

When Jesus Christ was being tried, he never argued or pointed to Barabbas saying, "Kill him, not me, I'm innocent!" Christ never fought back saying, "It's not fair, you people are sinners and shall pay for your evil doings." While Christ was on the cross He didn't complain or blame others for tattling on Him saying, "I can't believe Judas did this to me!" Jesus Christ knows the creation of all energy and, thus, He only created Godly energy. This example touches the heart of even the hardest of hearts and encourages us to change. He was pushed beyond imagination and yet He naturally forgave His accusers and His abusers; in fact, He never even needed to forgive, because He never held a negative feeling in the first place. This is our goal, to be like Christ and to be able to live the higher law as He did.

Let's be real here. We do not expect us all to respond Christ-like all the time. Because we are imperfect, we need to plan ahead before the conflict becomes too messy. Preferably before the resulting behavior creates havoc in your relationships. What are some ways to break the cycle when you are slipping into the role of the victim? Most preventative measures are far better than clean-up in the midst of drama. However, tapping helps balance the hormonal reaction, making it easier to think through a shift in the automatic reaction.

~~~~~~

Self-Care

Self-care can be the first step in prevention. This can include meditation, affirmations, and energy work. We all know it feels selfish to take care of ourselves first, but if we delay our own needs too long we drown in the needs of others with no strength left to serve. We have all heard the popular saying "put on your own life jacket first," but do we truly incorporate this into our lives? Everyone is different, no two people will experience self-care the same. The purpose of practicing self-care is to gain clarity of your needs, figure out where your path in life is leading you, to become passionate about who you are, to gain confidence and to take a "time-out" for your needs to build up endurance for life once again. Some examples of self-care are: sleeping in, attending a support group, a massage, a bath, a quiet prayer, running, walking, shopping, service, putting on make-up, watching a movie, reading a book, reading the scriptures, drawing, playing with the kids, talking to a friend, kayaking, swimming, being alone, sewing, crafting, cleaning, organizing, etc. Switching up your self-care is important too, because if you watch a movie or go for a run several times a week, it becomes a routine and is part of your lifestyle. And the point is to have a break from your lifestyle.

What does self-care look like for you?_____

_____

_____

_____

_____

~~~~~~

Negative Cords

Negative cord with others: These can be either converted into positive cords or removed. Converting cords can offer healing with the potential of improving relationships. All negative cords between a client and all others can be address at the same time. Examples of how to convert and remove are provided below. The first example (converting) is provided within the context of a family. The second example (removing) is in the context of all individuals that the client has negative cords with.

Convert negative cords between spouses or parent/children relationships. Negative cords with family: Bring to light all negative cords and rebellious spirits upon these cords and remove them. In the name of Jesus Christ command all rebellious spirits to depart from these cords and then seal all portals. Close your eyes and imagine negative cords with your family members, each created due to an event or misunderstandings or conflict. Choose to follow the lead of Jesus Christ and shine LOVE into each of these cords; such Christ-like love that all the negative energy within the cords is converted into healthy, healing, forgiving and loving cords. Continue shining this light until all negative cords have been converted.

Remove negative cords with others: Bring to light all negative cords and rebellious spirits upon the cords and remove them. In the name of Jesus Christ command all rebellious spirits to depart from these cords and I seal all portals. Detach all negative cords with all others. Cut these cords with the Sword of Forgiveness or dissolve them with Christ-like brotherly love. Release and remove the cords. (You may need to release some dark energy and/or traumas to fully keep these cords from reforming due to pain that is still present.)

~~~~~~

Assignments

Energy Work:

1. Do another dark energy release and/or the translucent energy.
2. Increase shields: Property shields, love shields, body armor, basic shields, truth shields, sound proof shields, invisibility cloak shields, etc.
3. Continue working on infections, toxins and food intolerances.
4. Continue increasing food/water/home vibrations.

Homework:

1. Practice self-care daily, a few minutes or longer each day. Commit to daily self-care throughout the rest of this program while working these steps. Notice if you find more energy or if you start to develop new talents. Notice a shift over time where you feel more positive and life has more meaning. You will have more to give when you have taken care of yourself first.
2. Continue daily affirmations for the next 90 days: test to add any that are needed.
3. Complete the automatic thought response worksheet if not completed during the session.

Self-Sabotage

Step Five

Clear Your Space

Test your client to see if these steps need to be completed before continuing. These steps are found in the Appendix. Always begin your appointments by checking for "attacks."

1. Begin by clearing the space and removing all dark influences/rebellious spirits
2. Remove Self-Destructive Tools of Dark Influences
3. Remove Mind Subconscious suggestions
4. Remove Intimidation Energy
5. Ask for shields of protection

~~~~~~

Enjoy the Ride

There was an interview between a motivational speaker and two musicians. The musicians were asked the same question, "Do you enjoy speaking or performing in front of an audience?" The first individual said, "I hate it. I get this knot in my stomach, adrenaline pumps through my body and I get so anxious… It's horrible." The other individual responded to the same question with exhilaration in his voice saying, "I love it. I get this knot in my stomach, adrenaline pumps through my body and I get anxious and so I use that excitement to propel me on stage to change lives." So what's the difference between these two experiences? It's all in your perspective – **your attitude and your perspective define your reality**. At first I thought this was just what talented people say to the rest of us, while being full of bologna. But this is a message of agency, just spoken in different lingo. Sometimes we feel powerless to the events in our lives, sometimes we make mistakes, but the difference between someone who sees trials as miserable and someone who sees the very same trials as gifts is simply by utilizing free will and shifting their perspective.

I would like to share a story with you. I chose to load up my oldest daughter and drive to an amusement park, slather on sunblock, pay an arm and a leg and ride roller coasters all day. When I came to the first ride it was the boat swing. A very simple ride. I sat down and the boat starts to swing … higher and higher. At the peak just before dropping I felt the all too familiar sensation of DREAD. My stomach rose in my throat, I felt like I might pee my pants, and I felt completely out of control and I hated it. I told myself, "I don't want to be on this ride, I don't want it to drop, and I don't like this." At the same time, I was praying the ride would casually stop and let me off. BUT at that moment I remembered something I had learned – it's all in my head, it's all my perspective, and it's all how I talk to myself; change the inner dialogue and change the experience completely. As a test, I chose to shift my thoughts and see if those crazy people knew anything about what they were talking about. I said to myself, "I'm safe! I chose to drive here, pay to get in, stand in line and climb on this ride for the main purpose of this very sensation of a thrill; therefore, I am fully in control of my choices and actions. This is FUN! I am having the time of my life and I'm just going to enjoy the ride, I do not wish to change it in any way." Guess what? I experienced something I've never experienced before. I did not feel my stomach rise in my throat, I did not feel like peeing my pants, I did not feel out of control. I did not feel anxious to get off, in fact I threw my hands in the air and just let go! I felt this beautiful connection with myself and the ride was fully enjoyable.

For the first time I enjoyed the ride! So I chose to test my new found experience on a very steep, intense coaster. I had to give myself a pep talk the entire time going up the steep grade. But letting go of control and enjoying the ride was an experience that stayed no matter how scary the ride! So before leaving the park we chose to really challenge my fear of heights by riding the sling shot/bungee/sky diving ride. It's a ride that straps you in as a single or double rider in a body suit and drops about 100 feet while swinging you across a lake. I've always been deathly afraid of this ride and I chose to test myself with an extreme fear by using my new perspective shift of "It's all inside me." My daughter and I were raised higher and higher and higher still. I grew excited and nervous, but continuously fed myself positive encouraging thoughts of optimism and safety as I had done before. I pulled the rip cord and we dropped the 100 feet and my excitement grew as did the sense of FREEDOM. I was alive for the first time flying through the air without a care in the world, living completely in the moment!

You see, the roller coaster ride is the exact same ride it had always been, the ride didn't change at all! The ONLY different was MY perspective. I think this experience gave way to a whole new perspective towards my entire life. How often have I tried to control the outcome or have controlled my experiences due to fear of everything or everyone, which I have no control over. How often have I chosen fear over LOVE? How often have I changed my experience, because I was afraid of the outcome? Is this the life I wish to continue leading? The entire shift is within ME! I wonder how different my experience in life would be by just shifting my perspective and just choose to "enjoy the ride?" It's all inside me. I can choose every second of my life by the way I perceive my circumstances. Every day we get to choose who we are and what we want. Every choice shows where my priorities are. The past does not equal the future. My history doesn't hold me hostage. TODAY is a new canvas to paint. So how do I want to show up in my life? My external world is a reflection of my internal world. You could choose to enjoy every second of your life and just enjoy the ride. The only thing you can control is YOU! Letting go of the outside control factors is the shift we will take today.

Filters

When we experience an event, our memory of that event is filtered through our perception of the world and the individual(s) involved. Energy is formed around the events throughout your past experiences and the manner in which they influenced you. We store this energy, because our subconscious remembers events through our emotional memory. My memory of an event may be vastly different from the manner in which you remember an event. This perception is created through our core beliefs, our self-talk and **our assumptions**. Most likely we think we misunderstood events or another person; therefore, there's always a chance that our emotional memory is not 100% accurate. When we recognize this, we choose a healthier perspective, a more loving and forgiving perspective for others that we share our lives with. With this energy release, we are only beginning this shift by releasing the negative energy that we have held onto for all these years and slowly beginning this shift into a healthier mindset for the future. This mindset will bring us closer to living the example set by our loving savior, Jesus Christ.

Everything we experience holds an emotional memory within your body. You can think of something emotional from 10 years ago and still feel the pain and heartbreak of the event just by remembering the event. As we release the negative energy of that event, you will be able to remember the event with a more rational understanding that is free of reliving the emotional trauma. Most memories are emotional and when you perceive your past with a new and more Christ-like perspective that is free of the negative energy, you are free to rewriting a new story for your life, who you are and how you perceive the world around you. Remember your thoughts have power!

Visualization: There is a hurricane within you – your spirit, mind body and energy fields. This storm is creating chaos with your negative energies, memories and thoughts with all sorts of dark experiences flowing around in complete chaos. It is time to settle this… slow it down into a wind and then a slight breeze. Now you can begin to identify some of these negative thoughts and energies and what they are. Now slow it down until it begins to fall. Allow it to fall to the ground. You can now see that there are faulty core beliefs, limiting beliefs, negative filters and blocks within your spirit and mind. There are also walls, veils and such, to protect you. There are many different energies and components that have fallen to the ground. Shine the light of truth and knowledge upon all this mess – shine it upon the core beliefs, limiting beliefs and the filters and allow the light of Christ to filter out any misperceptions so you know deeply within you the nature of all things. Allow your mind to identify those that are of a Godly nature and those that are of the adversary. Consciously choose to reject that which is not of God.

As you see all this negative energy, faulty core beliefs, limiting beliefs, negative filters, blocks, walls, veils, memories, thoughts and all other components on the ground it starts to flow downhill as if on a mountain. This downhill course is the loops and thought processes associated with all of this. As it flows downhill it starts to flow into small streams and into a large river. It eventually flows into a canyon full of negative energy… All these energies that flow deep within you has only one path to flow into and it doesn't flow out and it leads to ill health and death. It is very limited. If you were to stand at the bottom of the valley, it would seem impossible to get out of this valley. The negative energy only knows this one route.

Now take your hands and push this valley together; push it together and bury it all deeply within the earth. The earth is healing. Over time, it will convert all the negative energy that was within this valley – all this energy, the beliefs, filters, blocks, walls, veils, memories, thoughts, loops, cords and components. It is now all buried and as the earth converts this energy your spirit, mind and body may distribute the positive energy to where they like.

Now imagine all of the positive energy flowing all around you: peace, love, confidence, stability, calm, forgiveness, wisdom, optimism, rejoicing, etc. Invite this energy into your spirit mind and body. Allow it to flow into you. Now let that positive energy rain down upon your ground and let it start to trickle into a small stream. Follow it down into a big river and allow it to flow into a large valley. In this valley and river – it all has positive core beliefs and positive filters. When a negative energy comes in – it is filtered right out and converted into positive energy. This valley is beautiful, lush, filled with wildlife, fresh air, and energy to your soul. This isn't the only valley you have – you have innumerable valleys similar to it. The energies are not trapped and it can easily move to any valley it desires. The valleys do not come to an end within you. Let these valleys fill your soul and let them flow out of you and into others. Again, allow this valley to flow out of you continuously and provide healing to all others. Take a deep breath… and let it out. This ends the visualization.

~~~~~~

Your Story

"Many of us are slaves to our story, a disempowering story that happened to us or something we did that we can no longer control. The story lives on in us in our language, in the way we replay it in our mind's eye like a movie. Replay it in a deliberate way until the mind and body know you are in control of the story. Replay it in the head with different colors, faster, different soundtrack, backwards, forward... Modify the story to help one feel in control, so you aren't terrorized by the story as it plays back out of control. When we replay a scary story in our heads, we put ourselves in the middle of the story as if we don't know how the story ends… but the truth is we do know how it ends." – Taken from the Tony Robbins Strategic Intervention program.

Everything we experience holds an emotional memory within the mind and body and spirit. If you haven't your past, you can think of something emotional from 10 years ago and still feel the pain and heartbreak of the event just by remembering the event. As we release the negative energy of that event, you will be able to remember the event with a rational understanding free of reliving the emotional trauma. What is your past story? Meaning, if I were to ask you – who are you, what has your life looked like so far and where are you going, what is your response? What has been your story?

_____

_____

_____

_____

_____

_____

Most memories are emotional and when you perceive your past with a new and more Christ-like perspective, free of the negative energy, you are free to rewriting a new story for your life. This new story is about who you are and how you perceive the world around you from God's perspective.

What would your ideal story sound like if you had the chance to rewrite history and the chance to create a new future for yourself? Can you see the gift in the trials of your past? This life is a gift from God. The past is over, you are no longer the person you were 10 years ago. What a blessing! The mistakes you or others made were teaching tools and opportunities to improve or forgive. The past contained many joys and many struggles; however, do you see these struggles as heartbreaking or a blessing? Can you see the blessings in your trials? Can you begin to change your perspective so that the past feels like an opportunity to progress?

Every day we get to choose who we are and what we want. Every choice shows where your priorities are. The past does not equal the future. Your history doesn't hold you hostage. TODAY is a new canvas to paint. How do you want to show up in your life? What changes are you willing to make to see new results? Then feed your new belief system by taking immediate action. Think, speak and act as if this new belief is actually your current reality! This takes daily effort as this shift will not occur subconsciously. You are the creator of your own life. Step into your power and make this change for yourself.

Rewrite your internal blueprint. Your blueprint = what you believe you deserve. Your self-image is a creation that you have the power to change. You believe 80% of your self-talk and only 20% of what others say. Your brain is constantly seeking to be validated for the existing stories. So let's begin by discussing your story. For example if my past story sounded like, "I grew up in a poor part of town, I was overweight and sick. I learned that I was never safe and I would have to fight for everything I had; therefore, I learned I cannot trust anyone and life is hard. Nothing comes easy for me. Sometimes I lose my temper or fall into depression, because of how difficult life can be." Then the new story with a Godly perspective could be, "I learned at a very young age how to work hard. I do not take for granted all of the blessings in my life, because I know what it felt like to be poor. My parents did the best they could and I know they loved me even if they made mistakes. I feel gratitude for a warm bed, food in the fridge, and a roof over my head. I'm so grateful for those trials in my past, because I am a better person, I am stronger and I know I am safe, because I have created a safe dynamic for myself in my adult life. I know I am valuable and my voice speaks kindness to all. My past created me into who I am today and I love myself. I am a child of God." The difference is the second story may be written by someone desiring this new life. Maybe they are not experiencing this new story yet, maybe they are still living the first story, but this second story is the dream for a better life. Therefore, they begin to speak it as truth. As this occurs over time, you will become what you believe about yourself. When speaking this new story every day, you will then visualize it daily and then you will begin living it. You will begin making small changes daily to align your life with this desired lifestyle. When I wrote my story and my vision board 3 years ago, none of my story was what I was experiencing: however, after a year an amazing thing happened. I read my vision board and had an "aha" moment – my vision board was a direct reflection of the life I was currently living! I decided to update my story to expand my life even further. This is the most rewarding experience of personal development. I desire this for all mankind. So let's work together to rewrite your story:

Visualization: Close your eyes and envision yourself walking along the beach. The sun is setting and casting a beautiful hue upon the waters. Look off in the distance and see a figure dressed in white walking towards you. Listen to the sounds of the tide crashing into the shore and breathe in the fresh smells coming from the ocean. Become present in this moment and breathe out all worry or stressors of your daily life. Pick your own time of day in which you are walking and feel the temperature in the air as it reflect that time of day. You can even smell the salt in the air.

Focus on your breath. With each breath in, invite positive loving thoughts to flood your mind. With each breath out, breathe out the worries and stressful thoughts of your day. Allow the full vision of the event to flood your mind and senses. Leave your cares upon the beach. Continue releasing any stress, worries, negativity and leaving those cares upon the sandy beach as it is not beneficial to continue carrying them. Return your glance to the figured that is getting closer. It is a man; although, it is still unclear to you "who" he is.

Across the sky flashes scenes from your life and in those same areas below are written stories in the sand of what you've learned from those events. Some of the stories are positive while others are painfully negative. Some of the events in the sky are hard to witness and the learned story written in the sand is twice as painful as it affects your current life and your expectations for the future, so much so that you turn away from them. But you are tied to them and it is only a matter of time until you face them again. I invite you to take another look at the stories and ask yourself some questions. What is giving these stories power? Why does the past still hold onto you with such negativity?

Energy work: There is a rebellious spirit contracted to this old story. Bring to light the rebellious spirit and his contacts and his cords/chains. Command his contract to be given to you and wash it in the living waters or burn it. Then detach his cords/chains, cut them with the sword of limited freedom, release and remove the cords/chains. Offer him 3 choices: 1) Repent and become an angel in training 2) Depart 3) If you choose to attack you will be cast out. If he chooses to attack cast him out in the name of Jesus Christ.

Bring to light all frequencies (F) and vibrations (V) of the "old story" within the spirit, mind and body. Command all F and V of the "old stories" being held within the spirit, mind and

44

body back into a portal and seal the portal. Detach the cords connected to the old story. Cut those cords with the Sword of Truth. Release and remove the cords.

Back to the visualization: Now look at these stories written in the sand and recognize that these stories are solidified. Think about how easy it would be to rewrite them. Invite a large wave from the ocean to come in and wash away the story on the sand.

The man from the distance is now close enough that you can instantly recognize Him as the Savior. He approaches you and holds your hand while offering you His complete love, expecting nothing in return. Ask Christ to assist you in rewriting your story about yourself. Ask Christ to show you your worth and your potential. He smiles and across the sky flashes scenes from your life that have yet to occur. Amazing scenes you never thought were possible ... every dream being lived ... your ultimate potential being a reality. He offers to help you rewrite your story from His perspective; a story that is filled with hope, love, compassion, forgiveness, understanding and progression. Christ places His hands over your eyes and removes a filthiness that was clouding your eyes and causing you to see clearly. You are now able to see your own potential and rewrite your own story about yourself. Thank Christ for His constant love. Ask Christ for His staff and begin writing a new story into the sand. This story can change and grow as you progress, it is never solidified. It is ever changing, ever growing and ever improving. There are no limits, no bounds. You are capable of creating anything you desire simply by shifting your interpretation. Open your eyes and begin writing this new story. Listed below are some topics or areas of your life to focus upon when rewriting your story.

1. Spiritual relationships

   _____

   _____

2. Relationship to self

   _____

   _____

3. Relationship with others

   _____

   _____

4. Health

   _____

   _____

5. Wealth

_____

_____

6. Contribution

_____

_____

~~~~~~

Life Vision / Conscious Lifestyle Design

You must gain clarity of exactly what you want before seeing it manifest in your life! Let's get detailed here, please take this assignment seriously and truly see this as an investment in your future. All it takes is some time and effort. You are the one creating your life and your future. I recommend you invite God into your story and allow the true purpose of life to drive you. Yours will look nothing like mine. We are all very different, seeking different purposes. The more you become familiar with yourself, the more you can become passionately motivated about your life.

We are going to create a vision board with 9 categories listed below. If you can visualize it, you can create it! You can use pictures and write on a poster board or write a blog or a journal, detailing your vision. However this looks to you, take responsibility for the results in your life by focusing on the vision you have created for your future. Stay **vision** focused and **passion** motivated! Write these as if you are already living them as truth. The next time we talk, I would like you to share this vision board with me so we work together towards aligning your life with your goals.

1. Love Vision
2. Reputation Vision
3. Wealth Vision
4. Spiritual Vision
5. Family Vision
6. Travel Vision
7. Education Vision
8. Achievement Vision
9. Health Vision

Example: In my life I was newly divorced, sad, lonely, overwhelmed and the weight of the world was heavy to carry. I was in every support group and personal development seminar possible to help me to overcome my trials. Here's a snip-it of my vision board:

The 'LIFE VISION' is a compilation of what I want out of life. Victimhood is a result of wandering around through life, lost in an array of confusion, never "finding" happiness. When I know where I am going, what I want out of my life, where I am currently and how to get to my destination – then I am fully capable of living mindfully in the present.... completely content in

46

the moment and living as a CONSCIOUS CREATOR of the life I want to live. So when we break down our beliefs and dreams and desires for ourselves into 9 categories, we can explore and continuously grow in the right direction. The following categories are my personal belief system and an explanation of where I choose to put forth my energy and what I want out of life. This list is ever changing as I grow and learn. I am writing this proactively, so even if there's a category I struggle with, it's written in a way that I am NOT setting myself up to fail. Instead, I will succeed as I already have in so many ways.

Love Vision – The scriptures tell us to "Love others as thyself," but how can I truly love someone else until I love myself? How can I allow someone to love me; if I don't believe that I deserve to be loved? My love tank is full when I love myself and I'm filled with God's love. Therefore, I am not seeking outside of myself for acceptance, love, or happiness. I believe I am a whole person, so I am looking for another whole person (not my other half) who already loves himself and has God in his heart so that together we can be growth partners. God is preparing me for something amazing. I will utilize this time to grow and prepare myself as a more patient, more loving woman who can communicate better and I will be emotionally healthy enough to bless and serve the man of my dreams. I choose to treat him as my King; therefore we fill the air with a sweet aroma of mutual respect and Christ like love. I will become the person I want to be with, and then I'll attract that kind of person naturally. I choose to respect myself and see the beauty within instead of the temporary flaws of my flesh. I see myself in the same light as my Father in Heaven sees me. I deserve so much more than I have ever experienced and one day, the right man will see the beauty inside me and choose to spend eternity by my side as best friends and live out our days without contention, instead filled with peace, love and joy. I am not disposable. I will not allow men to treat me as though I am. I am worthy of Love and Belonging. My heart is a treasure and I will only share my heart with those who earn it. I am beautiful inside and out. I will only allow men in my life who treat me like the Queen Heavenly Father created me to be. I love myself! Be the Goddess you were destined to become and be worthy of the righteous man you seek.

~~~~~~

Assignments

Energy Work:

1. Release another dark energy. Always test and release the most critical.
2. Monitor specific needs for a compound.
3. Continue working on the treatment for toxins, infections, and food intolerances.

Homework:

1. Write your Life Vision / Vision Board with each category.
2. Work on your new story so it can align with your new vision for your life.
3. Continue daily affirmations and test for more. Place affirmations throughout the house for continual reminders.

Self-Sabotage

Step Six

Clear Your Space

Test your client to see if these steps need to be completed before continuing. These steps are found in the Appendix. Always begin your appointments by checking for "attacks."

1. Begin by clearing the space and removing all dark influences/rebellious spirits
2. Remove Self-Destructive Tools of Dark Influences
3. Remove Mind Subconscious suggestions
4. Remove Intimidation Energy
5. Ask for shields of protection

~~~~~~

Spiraling Gratitude

I would like to invite you to take a moment to focus on what you are grateful for. Sometimes it may be hard to see God's blessings or find anything to be grateful for when we are surrounded by turmoil. So let's do this together with a practice called Spiraling Gratitude. We begin inward and work outward starting with the most basic functions of life.

Begin by putting your hand on your heart and feel the heart within you beating and pumping blood through your entire body without any conscious effort on your part. This heart of yours works tirelessly night and day, 365 days a year for many years straight with no break. You do not have to tell your heart to beat; this is a gift from God.

Now focus on your breath as your chest rises and falls, filling your body with life giving oxygen also keeping you alive and working along with other systems to keep this body you are using functioning to the best possible capacity to sustain life.

Now focus on your skin and the sensations of what you may be touching at this moment. Touch is a temporary gift while we are experiencing a body of flesh and blood; it is a gift to be used wisely. Every part of your body can give or receive life giving or life draining touch. This is a powerful gift from God, let's thank God for trusting us with this gift and for the experience to see, feel, touch, taste and hear everything in life. Think of how lucky you are just to be alive with this body that God made just for you!

Now work outward a bit. Think of the meal you ate this morning and how easy it was to purchase and prepare, knowing how much work went into growing or making that food you purchased and offer gratitude for that meal that keeps you alive as some people in the world are starving. You are blessed to have food available in your home to eat and electricity to cook that food, all without building a fire first or foraging for food.

Now let's spiral out even further. Let's think of your lifestyle – you are in a country where religion is free and you can attend church, not to mention you are healthy enough to be alive today. We are blessed to have the restored gospel in our lives; this was given through many who sacrificed everything to bring us this gift. Not everyone has the luxury that you do to experience even the basic truths of the atonement of Jesus Christ. Think of your family, friends, job and luxuries. All these are gifts, regardless of how your life looks.

When a college professor gave his students a sheet of paper with a single black dot in the center, he asked them to describe what they saw. Every student described the black dot and its role on the page. Not one student noticed the 99% of the paper that was blank white. You see, we naturally tend to focus on what's wrong in life, this is to ensure survival, but it tends to overwhelm every aspect of life to the point that we cannot see the rest of the beauty surrounding us. When we consciously choose to focus on gratitude, we experience a different result. When we start seeing the gifts we live each day, we naturally want to share this with others and, thus, service is born. There are many who need your service and assistance as we are all brothers and sisters and our Father desires for everyone to receive His message – and this message is that of LOVE.

Mosiah 2: 19-22 "…O how you ought to thank your heavenly King! I say unto you, my brethren, that if you should render all the thanks and praise which your whole soul has power to possess, to that God who has created you, and has kept and preserved you, and has caused that ye should rejoice, and has granted that ye should live in peace one with another— I say unto you that if ye should serve him who has created you from the beginning, and is preserving you from day to day, by lending you breath, that ye may live and move and do according to your own will, and even supporting you from one moment to another—I say, if ye should serve him with all your whole souls yet ye would be unprofitable servants. And behold, all that he requires of you is to keep his commandments" (Book of Mormon)

God's Expectations

Most of us struggle with desiring the approval of others. How do we shift this? Whose approval truly matters? I believe we desire the approval of others, because they are our peers, our judges, our friends, our co-workers, our bosses, and our family. When we care more about the thoughts and opinions of others, we forget about our own opinions or thoughts. Is it worth ruining your own experiences to please someone else? Can you control someone else's thoughts or opinions? Let's talk about this. In the pre-existence when Heavenly Father announced the plan to come to earth and gain a body, there were two volunteers to be a Savior, Jehovah and Lucifer. Jehovah desired to follow Father's plan, but Lucifer desired everyone to return to heaven and succeed. So if you truly believe this occurred, then the desire to get everyone else's approval or worrying about other people's thoughts to the point of wanting them to think certain things about you is the plan of Lucifer. This means when you feel this way, you are not being influenced by the angels or the Holy Ghost. This changes things doesn't it? If someone is rude to you, how would Christ respond? If someone does not approve of you; how would Christ respond? Does He desire to change their minds? Or does He offer is everlasting love and do what is right with His own life, leading by example. The approval we need to focus upon is our Father in Heaven. What does He expect of you? What changes do you need to make in life to please him?

1. **Repent!** Stop sinning, not only in deeds, but also in thoughts. Practice all the atonement steps, including forgiveness, towards yourself and others. The healing that comes from praying for your enemies heals your heart quicker than expecting an apology. How do we respond to hate? There are many people destroying human life in the world. How do we forgive all our brothers and sisters? Christ taught us to forgive 70x7 and to turn the other cheek. When someone reaches out with hate and anger the human response is to respond with hate and anger... But that's not God's model. God responds with love, patience and forgiveness.

   > Matthew 5:38-44 Ye have heard that it hath been said, An eye for an eye, and a tooth for a tooth: But I say unto you, That ye resist not evil: but whosoever shall smite thee on thy right cheek, turn to him the other also. And if any man will sue thee at the law, and take away thy coat, let him have thy cloak also. And whosoever shall compel thee to go a mile, go with him twain. Give to him that asketh thee, and from him that would borrow of thee turn not thou away. Ye have heard that it hath been said, Thou shalt love thy neighbour, and hate thine enemy. **But I say unto you, Love your enemies, bless them that curse you, do good to them that hate you, and pray for them which despitefully use you, and persecute you.**" (KJV)

So God is asking us to respond with Love. Although it is one of the most difficult things God has asked us to do, it is also one of the most important. Loving those who love us is easy, but loving those who hate us, is a challenge. Mother Theresa, Ghandi and Jesus all believed they could change the world by their example of love and forgiveness. You don't fight fire with fire, you fight fire with water! Forgiving yourself can be harder still; begin by apologizing to your spirit. Your spirit knows the larger plan God has in store, when you sin or even participate in dark thoughts, your spirit mourns and suffers. Always apologize to others and God too. Always accept forgiveness, because you deserve it! Your purpose here on earth is to learn, grow, progress and to return to our Heavenly Father. He does not want us to continue suffering from the past mistakes or trials. Trials are just accelerated growth opportunities after all.

2. **Keep the commandments.** The 10 commandments are the most basic. Obedience, structure and self-discipline create freedom. Freedom from addictions, misery and the

entrapment of the adversary. Once obedience becomes a joy, you will begin to naturally start living the higher law. This is the focus with our program – to prepare ourselves for the second coming and learning how to live the higher law right now. Some people still struggle with the commandments, the law of chastity or the word of wisdom. Why are there so many rules? Father knows so much more than we do. He knows where true freedom comes from. It may feel restrictive to follow all these rules, but it actually brings about the greatest freedom. Most people, who grow a testimony from obedience, will also see the amazing miracles waiting to bless their lives. They will also avoid unnecessary heartache that comes from alcohol/drug/food addictions, debt, infidelity, STD's, unwed pregnancy, etc. Heavenly Father loves us and only asks a little from us; I say unto you – it's time to make a change. It's time to practice obedience and see how it changes your life. But let's take it to the next level; let's go beyond the commandments. Let's learn to live the way Christ lived.

I would like to share a story with you. I recently walked into a grocery store feeling fragile, but upbeat. It happened to be one of those days where everyone was shopping at the same time. The stress and anxiety radiating from everyone in the store affected me and I, inevitably, left the store upset just like everyone else. How would this be different if Christ had walked into the grocery store? I'm assuming He would have shared His love and positive energy with all those who were struggling that day. I'm sure He would have influenced everyone with His spirit so positively that everyone else would have left the store crying tears of joy and feeling the healing power of His love. I'm also assuming Christ would have been uplifted by the opportunity to bring healing to others. What a beautiful goal, to find ways to lift others when they are struggling instead of being dragged down.

3. **Take care of your body and love yourself**. As a mother, I desire for my children to love themselves and learn to take good care of themselves. I want for them to succeed and love life. I believe this is what Heavenly Father desires for us too. I believe this is the driving force behind all that He asks of us.

> Doctrine and Covenants 18:15 "And if it so be that you should labor all your days in crying repentance unto this people, and bring, save it be one soul unto me, how great shall be your joy with him in the kingdom of my Father!"

Have you ever considered that one soul might be your own? Father wants us to return to Him having successfully completed our time on earth. You have been created in God's image, your spirit and body are perfect creations of God and you are a divine celestial being with infinite worth. Learning how to love yourself is crucial to your own progression. When I was young I suffered from bulimia. I didn't even like myself. One day I had a dream. In my dream I had died after reaching my desired weight. I approached Heavenly Father feeling satisfied and proud of my weight loss achievement. He said, "You didn't become a mother; you didn't fulfill your mission in life. All that mattered to you is how others saw you. You forgot about how I see you. You died in vain, I'm disappointed in you." I woke up bawling and realized I would rather be fat and happy, than skinny and miserable. I decided to stop focusing on what others think and start loving the body God gave me. I decided to focus on what God thinks.

Taking responsibility for your choices and results in life will greatly improve your ability to find self-love, which is far more fulfilling than external sources. Can you comprehend how much He loves you and how much He desires you to love yourself too? There's so much to love. When you study a tapestry on the wall and place your nose on the tapestry so your eyes are staring at a few pieces of thread, can you see the whole design? Can you see your timeline from the creation of your spirit, all the way to the potential for your future? Heavenly Father can… But we can't. The worth of your soul is great in God's eyes. Look at yourself every day and say "I love myself as God loves me exactly as I am right now." Say this every day in every way. When you see your imperfections, when you see what needs improving and you see the miracle of your existence come together into one – you will see the beauty of what this life has to offer: the opportunity to make mistakes, to learn, to grow, to heal and to progress towards your celestialized self.

4. **Love others.** This step sounds easy, right? Once you learn how to love yourself, you can begin to love others the way they deserve. Well, it is easy to love those who love us back … But most love that we understand is conditional. Do you love those that "despitefully use you, and persecute you" as taught by Jesus. Some of the most brutal divorces began many years prior with a loving marriage. It is hard to love those who do not love us in return. Christ taught us about this simple lesson of love, which a basic principle of life, yet it is one of the most difficult to implement into our lives.

If we take from His example of how to love, it would be without condition, it would be a perfectly pure love; similar to the love of a parent for their child. Could you love a stranger or your enemy the same way you love your own children? Can you be that "Good Samaritan" who extends your love? Think of this from Heavenly Father's viewpoint. He has a whole lot of spirit children and He wants everyone to succeed and get along. He wants more than that; He wants us to love each other. We are, after all, all brothers and sisters. I know that feeling when my kids love each other, it is so heartwarming. He wants us all to succeed, but we must do so together and love is the ultimate path towards righteousness. **Christ's ultimate message in His ministry has always been love. Learning to love others as God loves us is the main purpose of life!** To do this, we must always strive to be loving in our thoughts as well, so we aren't judging on the inside and smiling on the outside.

5. **Serve others.** This is the next step in self-care. God answers prayers through other people. So when you feel the inspiration from the Holy Ghost prompting you to serve, He is asking you to bless another. Service is ever so healing to both individuals. I typically think service is too time consuming for my already hectic schedule, but when I make the time and serve, my problems tend to resolve themselves. The best way to find a reprieve and invite the spirit into your life is always through service. What are some ways you can serve someone else? I don't mean the usual list or lame answers, but what can you do today for someone else? Make a habit of one act of service every day for someone else. While serving them, remember to offer them love as Christ loves. Allow this love to seep deeply into your heart. Do not serve for recognition; serve in quiet for the right reasons of spreading the love of God unto all our brothers and sisters.

My favorite act of service is one I do with my kids. We gather up extra food and snacks from the pantry, an inspirational book, and a few juice/milk boxes and put them in bags, along with a sweet message such as "God loves you!" Then we place the bags in the car and as we are driving we look for homeless people on the side of the road that may be hungry. I almost always park the car and hand it to them with a great big hug. Loving touch can be more fulfilling than any money or food. Sometimes I ask if there's anything else I can do for them, but I always follow the spirit. A few days ago my son divided up his Christmas candy and put a pile off to the side. I asked him why he was splitting up his candy. He said, "This is for the homeless people so they can enjoy chocolate too."

~~~~~~

Emotional Freedom Technique (EFT)

Your life is a creation of your thoughts. Automatic thoughts steer the direction of your results. Those thoughts begin with your core beliefs about yourself. This all makes sense right? Seems so simple until a conflict occurs. So, what happens when a trigger immediately puts you back into a dangerous place and you are feeling rejected and victimized? What can we actively do while deep in the trenches of self-sabotage? You may recognize you are presented with a choice and feeling miserable seems awfully natural and comfortable. In this conflict, the body goes into automatic protection mode. It's called the fight or flight autonomic response. It is a primitive survival instinct where the brain activates the sympathetic nervous system and pumps adrenaline into the body when a threat is perceived. This is a primitive automatic response that happens so quickly that most are unaware this is even occurring within the body. Our rational mind becomes disengaged and we become hyper focused upon immediate short-term survival.

The trouble with this automatic response is, in our normal daily lives we can become triggered easily, making it difficult to balance out the hormones in our systems. Purging these survival chemicals by sending a signal to the cognitive brain tells our bodies that we are now safe. If discharged safely, we can feel empowered and more able to handle situations in the future while feeling secure. But if we do not discharge the trauma and the excess stress hormones, then the primitive brain freezes the event in the system. At this point, the hormones will have an overpowering influence upon the mind and begin steering the automatic thought process, which leads to emotional responses that can be triggered by a situation that was similar to the original threat. In this day and age we are triggered all the time and the body is constantly in this fight or flight response.

The emotional freedom technique (EFT), also known as "tapping," is a non-invasive, emotional version of acupuncture. Tapping can assist in balancing out hormones/chemicals by releasing those them from the body in the same manner they were triggered to produce – through a specific emotion. We tap on certain pressure points in a certain order, while relaying our intentions to the energy flows in our meridians. When we tap 3+ times upon these points while saying/thinking of a particular intention, we are communicating with the glands in the body to produce or balance out the hormone levels. Since the imbalance began with an emotional event, we will counteract the imbalance by communicating with the gland that is over/under producing hormones by stimulating it with positive words/thoughts directly linked to the imbalance. A list of tapping assignments is provided in the Appendix. Test for tapping sequences for your client to assist in balancing their hormones. Write your own sequence if needed. Note: there are more tapping locations including the feet, knees and abdomen; these meridian points will be taught only to our advanced students.

Shorthand lingo tapping points: 1) Sides of the hands. 2) EB – inside of the Eyebrow. 3) SE – side of the eye, 4) UE – under the eye. 5) N – under the Nose. 6) L – under the Lip. 7) C – Collarbone/Chest. 8) AP – under the Armpit. 9) W – Wrist. 10) H – top of the Head

1. First we begin by tapping on the sides of the hands. Either option is ideal:

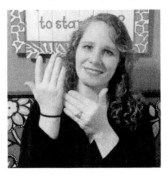 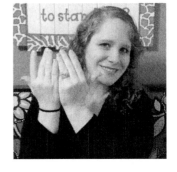

2. EB –Tap the inside of either or both eyebrows: 3. SE –Tap the side of the eye, on the bone:

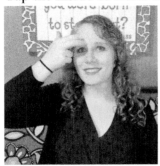 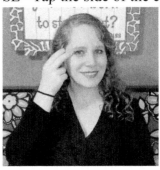

4. UE – Tap under the eye, on the bone: 5. N – Tap under the nose:

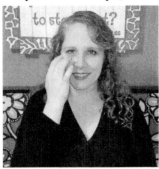 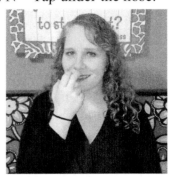

6. L – Tap under the lip:

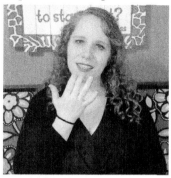

7. C – Tap the collarbone / chest:

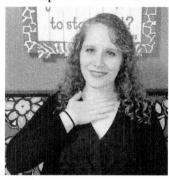

8. AP – Tap under the armpit:

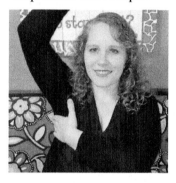

9. W – Tap on the wrist:

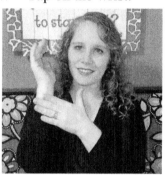

10. H – Tap on the top of the head:

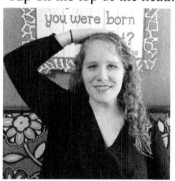

~~~~~~

Meditation

When we are overwhelmed with all the negative voices within normal daily lives, there are many techniques beyond affirmations. Meditation is a well versed method to center your chi. When doing this it may become difficult to control your thoughts and allow a space of complete positivity. Focus your mind on so much light and so much positivity that the darkness has no space to grow.

Be conscious of the words you pour into your mind and fill it intentionally with life giving words. When life giving words are constantly flowing through your mind, even in a high conflict situation, your thoughts will automatically feed your empowering core beliefs. Stand in your superwoman/superman stance, look at yourself in the mirror and with confidence say those life giving words. You can also voice-record them onto your phone and listen to them. Do this daily until your truly live them.

Below is a paragraph that you can use as an example. Rewrite the paragraph to be personal and special to you, filling it with your ideal affirmations and core beliefs:

"I am a royal child of God with infinite worth. I am the co-creator of my own amazing life, my life is a gift and I see beauty in my trials. I know my value, who I am, I know where I have been, and I know where I going. I deserve to have everything Heavenly Father has in store for me. I am healthy, every day and everyway I get stronger and stronger. I am surrounded by people who encourage me in my purpose. I love the people I spend my life with. My body is strong vibrant and energetic, I intentionally invest in my relationships. I live my purpose every day. I live in alignment with God and he pours blessings in my life, the past does not equal the future, the past is just stepping stones to a better future. My trials have become my triumphs, today I write a new chapter and a new masterpiece on this fresh canvas that is my life today. Today is a gift from God and I choose to live each moment to the fullest. I am a royal Child of God of Infinite Worth; there is nobody else in the entire world just like me. I love myself!"

Tony Robbins Meditation: We are not naturally wired for happiness. "We have a highway to misery, loneliness, stress, and a dirt road to happiness." – Tony Robbins. Let's wire your mind for happiness neurologically. To truly see lasting results in your life you must first practice daily meditation for 60-90 days to form new patterns. This is a guided thought process as it is nearly impossible to completely clear your mind of all thoughts. Do this meditation a total of 10 minutes first thing in the morning. Make time for yourself; wake up earlier or take your shower at night - no more excuses!

1. Explosive breathing pattern to alter your state
   a. Take deep breathe in the gut; in your nose and out of your mouth
      i. Do this 10 times; pause and repeat two more times (total of 30 times)

2. Think of these 3 things for 9 minutes and feel gratitude in each:
   a. 3 minutes – Think of something SIMPLE you are grateful for like the wind on your face or the smile of your child. Take pleasure in the simplest things in life, but be specific and truly focus your gratitude in your heart towards God's creations.
   b. 3 minutes – Imagine energy coming into your body healing every muscle, organ and strengthening every part of you. Then imagine every health problem being solved and answers coming into your mind to show you how to solve all external problems (that way you don't feel like you have to do it yourself). Feel this fully inside and out. Then imagine a circle going out towards your family and friends. Imagine that same energy getting to them; imagine them being healed, getting their problems solved, and having the life they deserve.
   c. 3 minutes – Think of 3 specific outcomes that matter to you. See, feel, and experience them as completed. Imagine the impact that it has in people's lives and feel that gratitude.

Power Hour

Now bring it all together: meditation, spiraling gratitude and life vision to create a "power hour." When we begin each day by feeding ourselves life affirming experiences and thoughts, we become emotional about our passions and blessings. These emotions will be more successful at creating new neuropathways for healthier dynamics.

1. Move your body.
    a. This helps your brain to function more efficiently in the morning.
2. Spiraling gratitude.
    a. As we practiced earlier – begin inward and work outward. Start simple.
3. Visualize your day and everything being successful
    a. Visualize yourself and others being successful in their endeavors.
4. Listen to your life vision
    a. Your daily thoughts will begin aligning with your life vision and your passion.
5. Speak/think your daily affirmations
    a. It takes 30-90 days to form healthy habits and thought patterns.

Assignments

Energy work:

1. Test your client for any dark energy or other needs they may have that are still restricting their progress or causing symptoms and complete these releases as needed.
2. Release and heal all destructive energy before continuing onto the next step.
3. Invite in positive energy into a fountain to be placed within their home to create continuous positive flowing energy throughout the home.
4. Refer to the charts in the Appendix for healthy and spiritual energies to invite into their meridian, test for the most appropriate ones.
5. Do a tapping sequence to balance the hormones in the body; refer to the Appendix charts.

Homework:

1. Practice the Spiraling Gratitude daily.
2. Write your own power hour affirmations and voice-record them on your phone; listen to it every day. Or write it out and put it on the mirror in the bathroom and read it every day.
3. Follow Tony Robbins daily meditation.
4. Make a 90 day goal and begin creating daily goals to align with this 90 day goal. It takes 30-90 days to create a new habit or thought pattern, so consciously practice improving daily habits. These daily and 90 day goals will be in alignment with your vision board to help align your daily actions with your desired results by starting with smaller steps.
5. Have an accountability buddy hold you to those daily goals.
6. Create your own daily declaration: I am statements or affirmations.

Self-Sabotage
Step Seven

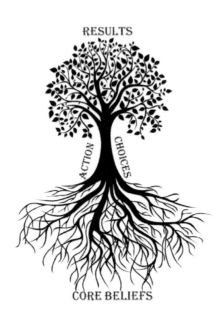

"I am responsible for the results in my life."

Clear Your Space

Test your client to see if these steps need to be completed before continuing. These steps are found in the Appendix. Always begin your appointments by checking for "attacks."

1. Begin by clearing the space and removing all dark influences/rebellious spirits
2. Remove Self-Destructive Tools of Dark Influences
3. Remove Mind Subconscious suggestions
4. Remove Intimidation Energy
5. Ask for shields of protection

~~~~~~

Tree Analogy

You are responsible for the results in your life. Your past choices create the result you are currently living. If you want to change your results then you need to change your current story about your life. The **roots** are your core beliefs. The **base** above the ground is the result of the seeds you have planted and created: your action and choices. The **leaves** and the **size** of the tree and the **fruit** are the results of your life. If you have a rotten apple – do you blame the apple or the roots? The roots must change to change the fruit.

Ask yourself, who would I have to be to naturally create my desired results? Examine your stories and how you came to this conclusion. We tend to live our lives staring backwards, thinking, "If people saw me differently, then my life would be better" or "If people really knew me, they wouldn't love me." We tend to focus on a faulty thought process of, "I'm not good enough because…" But the purpose of life isn't to escape problems or blame other people or situations; this removes accountability and any hopes for change as change requires awareness. The future is not going to be problem free either. Life hands us opportunities and chances; many can be viewed as accelerated growth opportunities. If you replant a new healthy seed, you can experience new tasty, juicy, delicious fruit and face life standing forward. The power is in the roots. Today we are going to do a core belief shift to help with the healing process that starts with the root system.

Organizing Core Beliefs

First we are going to reverse the core beliefs that are misconstrued – good is bad, bad is good. Healing = bad or sick = good. This can be more common than you know because the worldly view of healing can bring connotations of abandonment or hard work or fear of change. So we begin by acknowledging this learned mindset and resetting things into their proper location.

Energy Work:

1. Neutralize and defuse the Frequencies and Vibrations of all core beliefs.
2. Shine the light of truth and knowledge upon all core beliefs and allow the light of Christ to filter out any misperceptions so <u>the individual</u> knows deeply within the truth and nature of all things. Remind the core beliefs that which is of Heavenly Father vs that which is of the adversary. Consciously choose to reject that which is not of God and, therefore, train the body to no longer be tricked by the ultimate deceiver.
3. Detach the cords to the misperception and confused belief system
4. Cut the cords with the sword of truth
5. Release and remove the cords
6. Allow the core beliefs to naturally fall into their proper location and be seen for what they truly are. Invite in the spirit of love and faith in God for His plan for your life. Invite in your true self-identity as a royal child of God of infinite worth to resonate throughout your entire being.

Core Belief Conversion Preparatory Steps

Energy Work:
1. Invite the light of discernment to shine upon all core beliefs.
2. Invite all core beliefs to separate into 2 categories – faulty core beliefs and empowering core beliefs
3. Identify how many "original faulty core belief thought bubbles" the client has. (Identify the number)
4. Identify the number of "original empowering core beliefs thought bubbles" that is best for your client to convert the faulty ones into.
   a. List each original empowering core belief that is best for your client. (Make sure to only list the ones the client is ready to convert.) **This conversion will be completed below with a visualization, this is just the preparatory steps.**
      i. _____
      ii. _____
      iii. _____
      iv. _____
      v. _____
      vi. _____
      vii. _____
      viii. _____
      ix. _____
      x. _____
   b. Identify a color, an idea or an object to associate the new empowering core beliefs with. Add them to the list above
   c. Identify how many days the person needs to redo this visualization in order to solidify the shift.
      1. **Example:** 35 original faulty core belief thought bubbles – will take about three weeks to become fully integrated into their thought processes.
      Convert into 15 original Empowering beliefs
         1. God Loves Me – radiating white
         2. I love Myself – a rainbow
         3. I surrender my will and accept God's will for my life – radiating yellow
         4. I have faith in God – light of the sun
         5. I deserve unconditional love – royal purple
         6. I value experiences in life that offer growth – vibrant green
         7. Limitless amounts of energy flows through my body – red (deep blood red)
         8. God supports me in every step I take - earth brown

9. Positive Thoughts are powerful and empowering – sky blue
10. I find purpose in my existence – Deep yellow
11. I want to live – Double rainbow
12. I fully accept myself – soft pink
13. I choose to live mindfully in the present – lightning
14. I love and accept myself exactly as I am right now – valentine pink, red and purple
15. I move with ease through time and space. Only love surrounds me. – Sun, Moon and Stars

Preparatory conversation: Before beginning the visualization, it is important to recognize there is a problem – either you accept that the results are not desirable and that its belief is not currently serving you; or you choose to begin experiencing more connection in following the life of Christ and that you desire to heal the past. Seeing the truth in its real color will assist in seeing who created the belief in the first place. Typically the core belief begins small and gradually becomes bigger. When it begins, it is only mildly tainted, so mildly in fact, it is seen as harmless. By the end it is has become solid darkness and the strength increases tenfold. This is the way that Lucifer works to form faulty core beliefs. All this can be healed with a swift step towards God and a heartfelt desire to change. We are created in the sight of God, our bodies reflect His. When we look into the eyes of a child we are looking into the eyes of God. Technically, we are doing the same thing every time we look in the mirror, but a child is more lovable, teachable and accepting of praise. We can see a child's perfection and understand this analogy, but we'd struggle to accept it if it was geared towards us. Use this full understanding in your visualization, there is a level of choosing to accept yourself that must take place, a resolve to say – I love myself exactly as I am right now. Looking at yourself with compassion, mercy, and Godly love will bring much happiness unto you. Every cell within your body is created to lovingly care for you. Accepting your body, choosing to love it, then caring for it right back is the proper order to becoming one in body, mind and spirit.

~~~~~~

Core Beliefs Complete Conversion

Visualization: Close your eyes and imagine walking down the street. At the end of the street is a warehouse. It's large and it looks strangely familiar, you feel drawn to the warehouse doors and you enter in. As you look around you see _____ (number found in the above testing) faulty core belief thought bubbles. These are all different shapes and sizes and colors. Some are large like an elephant; others are small like a basketball. You have painted them all to look pleasant – as we all tend to paint the truth so it looks more pleasing to others. I want you to walk up to the nearest core belief "bubble" and press your face up to the bubble and look inside.

This bubble is filled with thousands of tiny bubbles and each of those tiny bubbles are filled with thousands of tiny bubbles. And inside each of those bubbles are thousands of tiny bubbles... Going on and on until there can be no more multiplication. This represents the thoughts within you. Each bubble contains an event that holds the emotions, thoughts and experiences that created it. Each within supports and solidifies the original thought bubble. Each original faulty core belief thought bubble represents a different event that created a whole new belief about yourself or the world. Your faulty core beliefs were created due to your experiences and therefore it is a learned belief that is deeply engrained for logical reasons.

Focus upon the bubble you are currently peering into, reach your hand inside this bubble and pull out a bubble which is an event that reinforced this original faulty core belief. I want you to inspect this bubble and tell me what event from your life are you holding? Can you see how this event contains many emotions and events and even relationships? Tell me what about this event was difficult for you and how do you believe it affected you in such a way that a faulty belief was created about your life?

Now turn the bubble around and study the event from different angles. I want you to stop looking at the trial for a little bit and see what happens… Look for a different perspective, maybe one you hadn't seen before; such as how this event has strengthened you, challenged you, or has taught you how to live your life differently. Can you see how Heavenly Father has blessed you and your family during this trial? Focus upon the blessings.

Now place the ball back into the main faulty core belief thought bubble. Take a step back to see all the bubbles within this warehouse and view how they are being hidden away from the world (possibly in shame). Ask Heavenly Father to completely remove the roof to this warehouse. Ask Him to let the sun shine upon this portion of your mind. As He removes the roof – the walls collapse outwards and all these thought bubbles receive sunlight for the very first time.

Look at the false paint job as it begins to peel off due to love radiating from the sun. Underneath you see the truth of the influences upon these thought bubbles. It is dark and deformed and not influenced by God. Ask for Heavenly Father to shine His love upon all these thought bubbles, the events and emotions within, so His influence is invited into these events and beliefs.

Now go up to that first thought bubble again and look inside, but this time do not focus upon all the bubbles within or the color of the bubbles. Instead, look THROUGH the main bubble and see an image in the back behind these bubbles. It is a scene from the pre-existence – of you and your Heavenly Parents. You are planning your life and choosing the events you would experience here, which will teach you and help you to progress. You chose these experiences for a reason and you agreed in advance to the events and trials that would occur in your life. Your choice remains intact and you chose to serve God even if others may exercise unrighteous dominion over you. All these events are for your own good!

Now I want you to look to your side and see Jesus Christ standing by your side. He is patiently waiting and offering you His perfect love. Ask Him to show you how He sees these events. Then ask Him the question, "What is my growth potential from these experiences from your perspective." Ask Him to help you to see the blessings you were offered through these challenges and help you to forgive yourself and others, so that true healing can take place and you can start to see your past from the perspective of Heavenly Father.

At this time, offer free will to these core beliefs – including the event, the actions of others, the emotions of others and your own feelings. This will allow a shift in perspective. This can be done through a personal prayer. Thank God for your free will; accept it and offer it to others. Understand God's plan and recognize that exercising control over others is a tool used by Satan. Recognize that taking control over our own thoughts and actions does not require us to take control of others' thoughts and actions. Remember to be slow to judge and swift to love and forgive. (Allow time for prayer to take place.)

Ask Christ to shine His light of truth upon all the original faulty core belief thought bubbles. Ask each original thought bubble to shine the light upon the inner bubbles and so on and so forth. Ask this light to shine forth a ray of sunshine, creating a brighter version of each.

A choice cannot be made until consulting with the past, present and future understanding of the world and what is best. The past offers foresight, when we change the view of the past and change the lesson learned from the past, it is oftentimes scary and takes a leap of faith. Being they were created due to a false understanding of fact, this light will assist greatly in showing the truth of God's creation. We cannot make a change that doesn't feel comfortable, safe or offer any foresight into the future results. This now rests upon the deeper relationship with God. This is good news; in fact, this is the best news ever! We have the support of God on our side. *Pause for a moment and ensure the light has permeated through all of the bubbles.*

Step back and look at all the original large thought bubbles and notice how their color is now lively and their shape more pleasant. Walk around and notice how each one is re-named into a positive empowering core belief with an associated color and representation. You will see the events stayed the same, but your understanding has changed – how you choose to see your past has changed. Therefore, the new empowering core belief is associated with these memories of the past, as God has been invited into these events to help you see the gifts in the trials.

These events have been converted from faulty to empowering with the love and light of Christ. I want you to walk up to the first bubble and see it has been converted into a new empowering core belief filled with memories and a new perspective shift reinforcing this new core belief:

1. Continue walking/inspecting each new original empowering core belief thought bubble and notice their new associated color/image one at a time (this is the preparatory list you prepared for your client, for example):
   a. God Loves Me: and the bubble shines with a radiating white
   b. I love Myself: and you see a beautiful rainbow coming from the bubble
   c. I surrender my will and accept God's will for my life: and the bubble is radiating yellow
   d. I have faith in God: and the bubble glows with the light of the sun

All of these thought bubbles now bring you joy and they are now free to roam, no longer being hidden within the darkness of a warehouse within your mind. Allow them the freedom to be seen, to be recognized, to teach and to learn. Now that they have each been converted, take a deep breath and let it out. This ends the visualization.

Positive affirmations: to reinforce the new empowering core beliefs. List positive affirmations by testing the best ones to use from the affirmations chart in the Appendix.

1. _____

2. _____

3. _____

4. _____

5. _____

6. _____

7. _____

8. _____

9. _____

10. _____

~~~~~~

The Nature of Emotions

The question may arise, who tempted Lucifer to turn to evil when he is the creator of such emotions? It was God who created all. Emotions can become much more powerful than their original creation, but God gave us all ranges of emotions to experience including jealousy, anger, revenge, sorrow, etc. However, it is God who teaches us to refrain from these emotions and the energy therein. Thus, Lucifer took all ranges of evil and expanded them into their maximum potential, but who creates these emotions within us? Is it Lucifer who tempts with anger or is it a natural part of our creation? A part that we are given to learn how to mature from and seek a higher understanding. Father would not give us only joy and happiness and then say, "You have agency, now go!" He offers us every emotion. Does this imply He also created pornography, sex trafficking, murder and cruel abuse? Father gave us the emotions, what we choose to do with these emotions are within our control. There is no angel tempting us to kill or take the life of others. This is why we have been given the 10 commandments. Likewise, the higher law incorporates this reality and increases the expectations of God until we deny all negativity that separates us from Him.

In the pre-earth life, we were aware of these emotions and how they would separate us from God; therefore, it was simple to refrain from the many temptations. Coming to earth posed a new set of complications as we did not know or understand the full measure of these emotions and how they would affect our mortal life. Imagine a child being fully conscious of all his actions and reactions with a perfect knowledge of his divine destiny. Do you think he would follow his own choices or would he pose in his perfections as he assumes the future role of his destiny? The purpose of explaining this is to say – we cannot understand the full reason why Father has offered agency, along with emotions ranging from Godly to sinful. But He does counsel us how to handle these emotions and how to love one another. This is why He sent His Son, not simply to die for us… This is a shortsighted answer. He sent His Son to live for us too. Christ taught us how to respond to hate with love. How to show love in the very face of evil, even when you cannot change the reactions of the evil placed in front of you. This is the basic understanding we wish for you to grasp… How to love even when the other person chooses hate and being okay with their choice. Why respond with anger when it simply breeds the exact thing we preach against? Sounds counterintuitive, but it is the natural response of many.

~~~~~~

Assignments

Energy Work:

1. Perform another dark energy release. Test for any further needs of the spirit, mind or body. Always be aware of further possibilities arising due to continued progression.
2. Test for any specific needs of the body, including a compound for healing energy.
3. Be aware of any concerns your client may be facing including fears and traumas. Do these energy releases as needed. Move on when they are ready. Always be aware of how fragile one may be during this changing process as their lifestyle is shifting, offer continuous support with a small support group if possible. Remember as life continues there will always be agency and trials. These energies we have released were created due to experiences; it's natural to recreate the past, but we are working to retrain the mind so this should be minimal.
4. Begin releasing trauma energies or sensory energies or addictive energies or sexual energies if any remain. The sensory energies include healing the RNA and the DNA as does the physical trauma so the body may still need these steps performed.

Homework:

Tap each of the new empowering core belief into your meridians daily to communicate with your mind the changes that have taken place. (Test for the exact number of times/days to repeat.) We are training the body to realign to the changes in the mind by communicating with the body to balance out the chemical reaction.

Self-Sabotage
Step Eight

Clear Your Space

Test your client to see if these steps need to be completed before continuing. These steps are found in the Appendix. Always begin your appointments by checking for "attacks."

1. Begin by clearing the space and removing all dark influences/rebellious spirits
2. Remove Self-Destructive Tools of Dark Influences
3. Remove Mind Subconscious suggestions
4. Remove Intimidation Energy
5. Ask for shields of protection

~~~~~~

Story of a Child

It is sometimes difficult to hand over a great burden to others. To assist you with this, I'd like for you to think of a child at the young and tender age of five. There are two scenarios here. What do you think you would prefer as the parent?

1. Your child is being bullied at school; however, he doesn't want you to know, because you might get upset or become burdened by his troubles or feel disappointed in him. The bullying progresses and he is beginning to show aggression at home. You don't understand what has changed, but your child is now pulling away from you emotionally as he becomes more and more isolated and depressed. You continue to wait, trying to offer him love, but he just doesn't see your efforts.

2. Your child is being bullied at school. He tells you about how his problem and asks you for help. You feel closer to your son as he leans upon you for comfort. He tells you how the other child is behaving and how it affects him. You see, it as a simple task to correct and assist these two young children. This is hardly a burden to you, as you desire to see the two kids enjoying themselves once again; in fact, the solution is rather simple. You teach your son ways to show love to this other child as they are struggling at home. Quickly, your son becomes friends with this other child and your son remains the happy child he has always been.

This scenario is similar to how our Savior can relieve our burdens. Too many times, we do not wish to burden God with our troubles, but these seemingly impossible burdens that we carry are a simple task for Him to resolve. His understanding is higher than ours; we are like children to Him. He takes pleasure in seeing us progress and learn from our mistakes. Allow Him to comfort you, embrace you and take this darkness from you while He expresses His great love to you.

Our Heavenly Father is pretty amazing. He offers us a list of rules to help us to be happy. He gives us counsel, the Holy Ghost, church leaders and the gospel. Jesus Christ takes our hand and even walks the path with us. He leads us in the right direction, but we tend to complicate things. Let's say you walk into a mall and check the map to route the way to your favorite retail. Jesus Christ nudges you that it's just a few hundred feet to the right and He offers assistance to get there. But we tend to say – No, I'm going to take the escalator down to the food court, walk to the exit, through the back alley, walk around the outside of the mall and then take the outside entrance to the store. Then the commute is exhausting, it starts to rain, and we complain that it's too hard, "Why me?" What's amazing is Christ never says, "I told you to take the easier way, you chose not to listen." Instead, He simply walks with us and offers constant love, support and still picks us up when we fall with a compassionate offering of constant love.

When Christ was on the cross He didn't say to his persecutors, "I forgive you for torturing me… Even though I did nothing wrong. I was just serving my brothers and sisters and obeying our Father in Heaven." He never expressed that He was being victimized or blamed someone else either. No, instead, Christ in His understanding of the larger picture simply says, "Father forgive them for they know not what they do." What an amazing example of love. This man experienced an automatic emotional reaction that was based on God's pure love in all circumstances. There was no negativity invited into His spirit, mind or body even in the most trying of times. What an example He is. This is my goal in life and I would like to begin living a more Christ-like centered life and I would love to have you join me in spreading this light of love that He has begun. So when Christ returns to the earth, He will see a world filled with light as we are living the message He taught. We can then welcome Him back to a world worthy of His presence. Let's spread this light by thinking as our loving Savior has taught us. The higher law was taught to us by the example Christ set. We must heal fully from the past so that we can change the course of our lives. Then as we change our patterns and habits daily, we will find over time we are ready for His return. We must begin now as time is running out.

~~~~~~

Alignment of Spiritual Vibrations

Do the following tapping sequences to assist the body after doing the Core Belief shift. The purpose of this sequence is to align the body's physical potential with the spirit's divinity. As we raise the vibrations of the mental state to align with the spiritual potential, we can begin shifting our perspective within the body's natural chemistry.

Reminder tapping points: Sides of the hands, EB – inside of the Eyebrow, SE – side of the eye, UE – under the eye, N – under the Nose, L – under the Lip, C – Collarbone/Chest, AP – under the Armpit, W – Wrist, H – top of the Head

"How Great Thou Art" EFT tapping – mostly taken from Stuart K. Hine's hymn

1. Tap the sides of the hands –
   a. O Lord my God,
   b. When I in awesome wonder,
   c. Consider all the worlds Thy hands have made;
2. Eyebrows - I see the stars,
3. Sides of the eyes - I hear the rolling thunder,
4. Under the eye - Thy power throughout the universe displayed
5. Nose - When through the woods,
6. Lip - and forest glades I wander,
7. Chest - And hear the birds sing sweetly in the trees.
8. Armpit - When I look down,
9. Wrist - from lofty mountain grandeur
10. Head - And hear the brook,
11. Eyebrow - and feel the gentle breeze.
12. Side of eye - And when I think,
13. Under eye - that God, His Son not sparing;
14. Nose - Sent Him to die,
15. Lip - I scarce can take it in;
16. Chest - That on the cross,
17. Armpit - my burden gladly bearing,
18. Wrist - He bled and died to take away my sin
19. Head - When Christ shall come,
20. Eyebrow - with shout of acclamation,
21. Side of eye - And take me home,
22. Under eye - what joy shall fill my heart.
23. Nose - Then I shall bow,
24. Lip - in humble adoration,
25. Chest - And then proclaim,
26. Armpit - "My God, how great Thou art
27. Wrist - Then sings my soul,
28. Head - my Savior God, to Thee,
29. Eyebrow - How great Thou art!
30. Side of the eye - How great Thou art!
31. Under eye - Then sings my soul,
32. Nose - My Savior God, to Thee,
33. Lip - How great Thou art!
34. Chest - How great Thou art
35. Armpit - Because God loves me this much,
36. Wrist - I too deeply and completely love and respect myself
37. Head - And all my brothers and sisters too

"I Stand All Amazed" EFT Tapping - Mostly taken from Charles H. Gabriel's hymn

1. Tap the sides of the hands
   a. I stand all amazed
   b. At the love Jesus offers me
2. EB - Confused at the grace
3. SE - That so fully he proffers me.
4. UE - I tremble to know
5. N - That for me he was crucified,
6. L - That for me, a sinner
7. Chest - he suffered,
8. AP - he bled
9. Wrist - and died.
10. Head - I marvel that he would descend
11. EB - from his throne divine
12. SE - To rescue a soul
13. UE - so rebellious and proud as mine,
14. N - That he should extend
15. L - His great love unto such as I,
16. Chest - Sufficient to own,
17. AP - to redeem,
18. Wrist - and to justify.
19. Head - I think of his hands pierced and bleeding
20. EB - to pay the debt!
21. SE - Such mercy,
22. UE - such love
23. N - and devotion
24. L - Can I forget?
25. Chest- No,
26. AP - no, I will praise
27. Wrist - and adore
28. Head - at the mercy seat,
29. EB - Until at the glorified throne
30. SE - I kneel at his feet.
31. UE - Oh, it is wonderful
32. N - that he should care for me
33. L - Enough to die for me!
34. Chest - Oh, it is wonderful,
35. AP - wonderful to me!
36. Wrist – God loves all His children so much
37. Head – That He gave us life
38. EB – He offers each one of us forgiveness through the gift of the atonement
39. SE – He gave us a planet to nurture us
40. UE – He created our spirit
41. N – He created our bodies
42. L – He offers us daily breath
43. Chest – Every second is precious
44. AP – every moment is a gift
45. Wrist – I choose to cherish this gift
46. Head – of a perfectly created body in the image of God himself
47. EB – A body that is unique as there is nobody else exactly like me
48. SE – I choose to use this opportunity I am alive
49. UE – To serve my fellow man
50. N – as my Savior has taught me
51. L – I choose to live my life the way He lived His life
52. Chest – I dedicate my life to serving the Lord and living the higher law
53. AP – I choose to experience righteous, holy thoughts
54. Wrist – of love for all mankind including myself
55. Head – Because I am a royal child of God with infinite worth

Resetting your Time and Understanding

Based upon the focus of our thoughts, we can live in past, present and future. We don't live one hundred percent in any of these time references; instead, we live a percentage in each. Additionally, we can live in the state of denial or a state of understanding. If you dwell upon these thoughts long enough, such as - remembering your past or daydreaming of the future, your mind will eventually drift towards living in those time references. The following steps will assist clients in resetting their time and understanding to a healthier balance of mindfulness.

Energy work:

1. Imagine taking a string about 6 feet long and placing it on a table. This string represents the timeline for your life. The far left of this string is your past. The far right of this string is your future. The center of this string is your present self. Now repeat these steps while visualizing this string being manipulated as such:
2. I separate my interpretation of the past from my current self. (Imagine picking up the left end of the string.)
3. I separate my fixed expectation of the future from my current self. (Imagine picking up the right end of the string.)
4. I reunite my interpretation of the past with my expectation of the future. (Bring together the left and right ends of the string.)
5. I separate this very moment into a space of suspended time. (The portion of the string in the middle where it bends represents the present moment.)
6. I shine a ray of truth upon my view of the past so I may more honestly comprehend the whole picture.
7. I trust my loving Savior with the future while accepting whatever may come with surety that with Him, all things are possible.
8. I now fix my attention upon the present moment and I observe the circumstances from a state of peace, quiet and solitude. I recognize and accept God's will and I align this very moment with His will.
9. I choose to live in the solitude of my choices and accountability. I choose to remove the outside circumstances beyond my control, as I can <u>only</u> control <u>my</u> actions.
10. In this space, removed from the past and the future, I trust fully in my Heavenly Father. I offer others the freedom to experience life of their own creation.
11. I remove myself from the limiting grasp of time.
12. I separate my clear and accurate understanding of the past and let go while allowing it to remain in the past. (Now place the left end of the string back onto the table.)
13. I separate the unknown, unlimited potentials of the future and release all expectations. I accept what may be. (Now place the right end of the string back onto the table.)
14. I choose to move forward living mindfully in the present.

Test before:	Test After :
% living in the past:	% living in the past:
% living in the future:	% living in the future:
% living in the present:	% living in the present:
% living in denial:	% living in a realm of understanding:

The Gift Hidden in the Trial

We remember things in fragments and we tend to focus on the worst parts. I would like to remind you that your testimony is strengthened when you are facing great turmoil, because we tend to lean on God 100% and this is where the true testimony is built. One day we will lean on Him 100% all the time, not just during times of trials. When we start to see trials as gifts... our perspective shifts and God's perspective is invited in. We are able to grow stronger as opposed to weaker or more defiant. We have the opportunity to turn to God in gratitude in everything we experience – from the breath you take, to the trials you endure. I am grateful for everything I have ever experienced, because it has created the strong person I am today, having found my voice and freedom. **I testify to you that - Your attitude and your perspective define your reality**. **When your perspective is focused on God, this will set the course of your reality**. We have seen such stories in the scriptures time and time again. I want you to ask yourself, "Where is my focus? Is my focus on the mistakes of others or myself for that matter? Or is my focus upon obedience to the teachings of Christ?"

How do we find the gift in the trial? It is not an easy task. I took the worst moments of my life and I used them, I challenged them, I educated myself, I found support systems and I utilized the atonement to help me forgive and heal, as I chose to move forward and learn from the past. I invited Christ into my life during the most humiliating moments and received the healing only God can offer. I am a better person for every trial. You see, this is similar to praying for your enemy. It sounds crazy to be grateful for the worst moments in life and our enemies, but when we focus upon the little bit of darkness we cannot see the light, but when we focus upon the light the darkness seems to fade away. Dr. Martin Luther King said, "Darkness cannot drive out darkness; only light can do that. Hate cannot drive out hate; only love can do that." Isn't that a profound statement? That is something to remember, not only in times of conflict with others, but when you feel that self-loathing feeling that forms dark feelings towards yourself.

When I was recovering from my divorce, I came across an amazing individual who was a very recent convert to my church, the Sunday after he was baptized; I sat by him and invited him to join me for dinner with the missionaries. I knew he was divorced and I knew how hard it was to attend church alone surrounded by families and couples; I assumed it might be particularly hard for a convert. I figured I could always use another friend and being I was rather introverted AT THE TIME, it was nice that he was passive and quiet. He was a very soft spoken man who I found out had read the scriptures cover to cover a few times already. WOW! Daily, we would study the scriptures together as he helped me to understand the lingo, which has been my stumbling block for many years. One day he asked me to begin a daily habit to pray for my ex. I admit I was shocked and a bit frustrated by this task, but I respected his wisdom and his experience. He calmly reminded me to make sure the prayer was sincerely asking for his happiness and healing. Over the course of a few months, this became a habit and it also became a testimony to me of how the Lord heals. I found MYSELF healing when I prayed for HIS healing. Using the scripture from Matthew again about loving our enemies, Matthew 5: 44, "But I say unto you, Love your enemies, bless them that curse you, do good to them that hate you, and pray for them which despitefully use you, and persecute you." This wise counsel is the foundation of the gospel of Jesus Christ and is a vital step towards living the higher law of Moses, where even our thoughts are pure and righteous.

Energy work: Compile a list of traumas your client has experienced with just a few simple key words. Do not spend too much time on this as we do not need much information and we do not wish to stir up unnecessary emotions.

Visualization: Close your eyes. I want you to imagine walking into a movie theatre and sitting down in a seat. The movie begins and it is a compilation of all the traumatic events in your life… Beginning with your childhood, then through your youth, your young adulthood and into your current stage of life. On the screen plays traumatic events that happened to you and to your loved ones, playing ONE at a time. These events play out in all their details as you watch helplessly from your seat in the theatre. It's as if you are right there experiencing them all over again. You feel anxious over how the events are occurring and you are even wishing to change the outcome, but feeling helpless and powerless as the events play themselves out on screen. You begin to cry into your hands as you experience the worst moments in your life all over again in their raw form.

Behind you a light begins to shine and as you peer over your shoulder through your tear filled eyes, you see the Savior approaching and He sits down in the seat next to you. His warmth fills up your space and brings much needed comfort as he reaches his arm around you to rest your head on His shoulder. You're not alone. And as the rest of the movie plays out, you are sitting next to the Savior. Through every detail, He continuously offers you compassion, understanding, safety, and love.

As the movie draws to a close after the last trauma ends, The Savior stands up and reaches out His hand to you to follow Him. He leads you down the theatre floor and up to the projection booth. Christ shows you the film from a different angle. He begins the movie of all your life's traumas… He simply smiles and explains this is for the best. You feel His peace and allow Him to progress.

You look down and notice you are still sitting in the theatre seats, alone, in a place where you are experiencing and watching the events as if they are still occurring. Although you are also in the projector booth with Christ. This time you can experience a significant amount of control over the event as you can change portions of the movie.

It is time to begin the movie, but this time each trauma has their own reel of film. Begin with the first trauma you can remember and watch it all the way through. You can speed it up or slow it down based upon what is happening and what you do not wish to see. If an area is repressed, blacked out or forgotten, this is God's grace as He is always protecting you. Take deep breaths and release the traumatic emotions with each breath. Remember you are safe now; this trauma you are watching is over.

Now make this trauma movie in a different color, but watch it backwards and in hyper speed. Then again forwards from the beginning. Watch this trauma play over backwards and forwards over and over as you control the speed and the color and even the narration.

Now look down at yourself watching the movie and communicate with yourself a message from the projector booth - what would that message be? What do you need to hear? Also tell yourself how these events changed you and how your family overcame these traumas.

Take the time to watch each trial separately one by one. At the end of each and every trauma movie, pick up the trauma movie reel and hand it to The Savior. Allow Him to relieve you of the burden of this trauma. Notice that when you pick up the first trauma movie reel, it may be hot, heavy, pokey or bulky. Watch when the Savior takes the reel, it is light weight and no longer burdensome, in fact you begin to feel gratitude for the events you experienced because you are growing stronger. What a blessing to be alive and experience all that life has to offer, including the trials as your scars are now signs of survival.

As you repeat these steps with each trial movie reel, interact with Christ and even invite angels to attend; your mother, father, grandparents, or other family members who may have passed on. Invite them to assist you and watch these trials along with you. There is no need to hide in shame, these angels love you dearly and desire your success. They fully understand your mortal life and the difficulties that earth life offers.

(Take as much time as necessary to continue through each trial reel until complete.)

Standing in the projector booth you look down at the entire movie of your life which is now playing again normally and you instantly are sitting back in the seats below with the Savior still by your side. You are surrounded by a circle of light from God, this light flows through you and all around you and this light is filled with immeasurable love. While you are watching the movie of your life notice that the emotions you are experiencing have changed. You are filled with gratitude and love. As the movie draws to a close and all the reels have been put away by the Savior, take a moment to say thank you to Christ and to the angels that have attended. Also say a prayer and thank God for your freedom and the gift that is your life.

Christ offers you a goodbye embrace and whispers this message into your ear. "Life is an opportunity to grow. Your perspective can shift to offer healing in moments where your agency has been removed. Your story is not over; use these trials to better yourself. Continue through life with your head held high seeking the gifts in the trials to better serve others. LIVE, embrace change, embrace growth, and embrace healing. You are never alone, I am ever present. Use your life and the time you have left, to bless others, be a sentinel of strength for others who are suffering. Reach out and use these experiences to bless others. Never remain lost; there is always a guide and an iron rod to lead the way. Open your eyes and open your ears to see/hear the guidance always being offered from a loving God. Remember your story is not over. There is so much more to write, so much more to experience, and so much more to offer. Use the experiences of the past to better yourself, to find strength and to bless your fellow brothers and sisters. My love is always with you."

Thank your Savior and say goodbye to all the angels who shared their love with you. Take a moment to allow the spirit to teach you of your own divine destiny and how to use your trials to create something beautiful with your life. (Pause)

Energy work: Bring to light all frequencies and vibrations of trauma energy in the spirit, mind and body. I convert all the trauma energy into this understanding, "I know I cannot change the past. I forgive all those involved in the traumas in my past as I offer a new perspective of understanding. I now see these traumas as a gift and a growing opportunity and for that I am truly grateful. I freely offer forgiveness as I choose to focus upon the gift of life that I still possess. I am grateful for the gift of free will that is given to everybody. I know I am valuable, I know I am a child of God and I know my existence matters. I am confident in myself and who I am. I love myself and I love this body that was created specifically for me. I accept that some changes have occurred due to these traumas and I offer my body love and gratitude exactly as it is right now. I stand all amazed at the love Jesus offers me; confused at the grace that so fully he proffers me. I tremble to know that for me he was crucified, that for me, a sinner, he suffered, he bled and died. Oh, it is wonderful that he should care for me. Enough to die for me! Oh, it is wonderful, wonderful to me! I marvel that he would descend from his throne divine. To rescue a soul so rebellious and proud as mine. That he should extend his great love unto such as I, Sufficient to own, to redeem, and to justify. I think of his hands pierced and bleeding to pay the debt! Such mercy, such love and devotion can I forget? No, no, I will praise and adore at the mercy seat, Until at the glorified throne I kneel at his feet. Oh, it is wonderful that he should care for me. Enough to die for me! Oh, it is wonderful, wonderful to me!" – I Stand All Amazed by Charles H. Gabriel

~~~~~~

Consciously Choosing a New Outlook

Visualization: Close your eyes. Notice a bunch of balls upon the ground. Pick up one ball and notice it is filled with potentials of a whole timeline for your life specifically. There are many balls, each with a different past and outcome. Let's imagine taking your current memories of your past, your current belief for your future and your current view of the present… And condense it all together into a ball that will fit into the palm of your hand. Take this ball into your hand and rotate it all around observing every aspect and crevice. Recognize the limitations within this ball. Place this ball onto the ground in front of you and walk away from it. Yes, walk away.

This life you are living is a gift from a loving Heavenly Father, a gift that is meant to offer joy and growth. Let's choose to explore and find another ball that will fit your dreams and desires for your life more fully. Keep in mind that your choices are endless. Amidst all the variety of options for your dreams and desires, see if another ball upon the ground catches your eye. Maybe a ball that is more glorious and bright and larger with a song playing from within. Recognize all the opportunities, freedoms, options and open doors available with this life you so desire. Pick up this ball and choose to unwrap the past, present and future to display a new existence. Now invite this ball into your life and place this ball within your heart. Invite the

74

ball's chakras to merge with your chakras. Invite the past to merge with your past. Invite the future to merge with your future. Invite the present to merge with your present. You are now surrounded by your dreams and potentials and the lovely song of this new life you have chosen for yourself. Take a deep breath and accept this new reality as it becomes "one" with your body, mind and spirit. Watch as this change expands to the edges of your new universe with a new understanding of the past, present and future. You can open your eyes.

~~~~~~

Merging a Couple

Energy work: Let's begin this topic on a very humanistic level. Starting at an early age, a man and a woman will seek out a companion. There is a natural instinct to connect with the opposite sex on a deep level that is beyond expression. Love… it makes you do crazy things, right? Young couples and newlyweds have a sparkle in their eyes, bursting with excitement and anticipation about life as they skip their way through life. Just as we have a physical compulsion to be with the opposite sex, our spirits have a strong desire to be connected with another spirit. Our spirits have the ability to make a deeper connection than what a physical body is capable of. Our spirits can literally merge with another spirit and form a complete energetic circuit between spirits. Merged spirits will offer one another their energy and strength in a synergistic manner, which in turn will offer each body additional strength. This is a sacred event and not to be taken lightly. When contention arises between merged individuals the spirits will disconnect for one another. After peace has been restored in the relationship, the couple can once again go through the steps to merge.

Couples can merge their spirits by following the steps below. The words need to be spoken by each individual.

1. Clear the Space between the individuals:
   a. Remove or convert negative cords (to include untying the knots in the cords)
   b. Remove walls/barriers/blocks
   c. Remove conflict lenses

2. Designate the space between each other as sacred and fill it full of love
   a. This can be done by simply statement such as, "I designate the space between (*name*) and (*name*) as sacred and pure and I fill the space up with love."

3. Merging: (the remainder must be stated simultaneously by each individual merging.
   a. Merging the 7 Energy Fields (MUST BE DONE FIRST in this specific order – outer most layer to the inner most layer):
      i. "I invite your (referring to the person you are merging with) **causal** field to merge with my **causal** field
      ii. "I invite your **celestial** field to merge with my **celestial** field."
      iii. "I invite your **template** field to merge with my **template** field."
      iv. "I invite your **astral** field to merge with my **astral** field."
      v. "I invite your **mental** field to merge with my **mental** field."

vi. "I invite your **emotional** field to merge with my **emotional** field."

vii. "I invite your **etheric** field to merge with my **etheric** field."

b. Merging spirits:

i. "I invite your spirit to merge with my spirit."

c. Merging Chakras:

i. "I align my chakras with your chakras"

ii. "I open my chakras"

iii. "I invite your chakras to merge with my chakras beginning with the root to the crown."

iv. "I invite our chakras to sing and dance." You can also invite them to engage in intercourse – yes, as crazy as it sounds, they will strengthen the bond between individual when this is done.

d. Combining vibrations:

i. "I invite my vibrations to combine with your vibrations."

Pep Talk

Continuously seek to improve yourself every day, but do not run faster than you have strength and do not remain complacent either. **As you are stepping out of your comfort zones, resistance will increase.** The people in your life are trained how to treat you and what to expect from you, so as you begin changing, they may resist. This occurred due to your previous lifestyle. Instead of allowing this to frustrate you, teach them how to support you, make daily small changes so the resistance is less intense. Be prepared in advance so the people in your environment will know what to expect from you. If you experience difficulty, offer yourself patience and love as the process is slow at times and takes daily effort to create lasting change. If you stumble, pick yourself back up and continue on your journey. The atonement is for everybody, as is agency, so we must accept that things won't always go the way we desire.

True change takes time, effort and patience. Take small simple steps that you can even do on your worst day. Creating a new habit or thought process takes 30-90 days of continuous effort before it becomes easy and natural.

Assignments

Energy work:

1. Test for the most critical energy to release with this step.
2. Create healing compounds as needed.
3. Continue releasing trauma energies or sensory energies or addictive energies or sexual energies if any remain. The sensory energies include healing the RNA and the DNA as does the physical trauma so the body may still need these steps performed.
4. Test for the most appropriate tapping sequence found in the Appendix.

5. Monitor food imbalances and hydration levels. We are creating a healing environment for the body and food can be healing or toxic based upon each individual body. Ask these questions and note the changes that have taken place:
    a. Is this good for me?
    b. Does my body want it?
    c. Can I digest it?
    d. Can I absorb it?
    e. Will this harm me?

Homework:

1. Pray for your enemies. Include those who cause you the most distress in your meditation visualization, where you see their problems being resolved and their happiness.
2. Tap in daily affirmations and the new Empowering Core beliefs from Step Seven.
3. Practice daily self-care and your power hour which includes meditation.
4. Continue with your accountability buddy to hold you to daily goals that are aligned with your life vision to help you reach your long-term goals.
5. Read or listen to your Vision Board.
6. Take daily accountability for your thoughts and words as they are reinforcing your new lifestyle, watch your self-talk and begin shifting in your affirmations as new loving self-talk.

Self-Sabotage
Step Nine

Clear Your Space

Test your client to see if these steps need to be completed before continuing. These steps are found in the Appendix. Always begin your appointments by checking for "attacks."

1. Begin by clearing the space and removing all dark influences/rebellious spirits
2. Remove Self-Destructive Tools of Dark Influences
3. Remove Mind Subconscious suggestions
4. Remove Intimidation Energy
5. Ask for shields of protection

~~~~~~

Your Perfectly Created Body

The body is holy and created perfectly by God. This holy creation is a temple for your divine spirit. Most negativity we experience becomes a natural way of life and you slowly become desensitized to it. Your brain has become trained as the neuropathways have formed thought processes due to your past experiences. As we are retraining the mind and healing from the past, it takes daily effort and patience. Many times, we may struggle with believing it is asked of us to live the higher law because of the difficulty of controlling our thoughts. When Moses was given the commandments with the higher law, he destroyed the tablets due to sin and the inability of the people to live the higher law. This doesn't make it any less important. By living the higher law, your Godly designed body will lead you the natural understanding that the higher law brings an alignment of health. Interestingly, Jesus taught us the most powerful healing tool in just a few short sentences. Matthew 22: 37-39 states:

> [37] Jesus said unto him, Thou shalt love the Lord thy God with all thy heart, and with all thy soul, and with all thy mind.
> [38] This is the first and great commandment.
> [39] And the second is like unto it, Thou shalt love thy neighbour as thyself. (KJV)

If a person fills their heart and soul with love for God and their fellow brothers and sisters here on this earth, there would be no room left for negative emotions. Yes, amazingly love is the healthiest pill a person can swallow. Love from God is the strongest form of love. A person can

78

invite into their spirit, mind and body the love of God. This can be done by simply stating, "I invite the Love of God into my spirit, mind and body." Adding to God's love, a person can also invite into their spirit, mind and body the light of Christ. These two positive energies are incredibly healing. We recognize that nobody in their mortal life is going to love perfectly, which in effect opens up space for negativity to reside within us. So, loving completely as Christ did is a lifelong goal.

When healing is focused in God and it is combined with the love you have for Him, this brings proper function to the body. This is because our bodies are created to function off of love. Wow, how powerful of a concept is that?... **Our bodies are created to function off of love.**

If we have a goal in mind and we focus on the desired result, it will lead to frustration. Instead, focus on the love of our Savior and everyone will be filled with a perfect love... A love that nobody can complete without Him. This love floods into the heart and the spirit and the mind and leaves no room for question or doubt of that love. To provide a visual perspective to this idea: Let's say our goal is to walk on water; how does one do that? Well, we do not walk on water by focusing by on the walking, because our minds do not believe we can walk on water. But when we focus on our Savior and his love we will find ourselves walking on water.

I'd like to explain another thing about love and that is: **Every negative behavior is a cry for love.** When we respond to a negative behavior with discipline, we are looking at the symptom and forgetting about the cause. Keep this in mind, when your enemy slings mud at you, he or she is merely seeking to fulfill a void/absence of love. Whether they realize it or not, they are literally begging for love and don't know how to express it in a healthy manner.

I'd like for you to consider something that may initially sound strange to you. I want you to look at your belly and say, I love you. Now, why in the world would I ask you to do that? Well, when any negativity is experienced, the body will react with an unpleasant symptom as it is toxic to the body. For many, myself included, we store negative emotions within our fat cells. **Those fat cells were created to protect you. Be grateful for them; show them your love and gratitude... seriously.** They hold energies of severe disgust and humiliating emotions, they have been surrounded by misery **specifically to protect you out of pure LOVE for the Creator** and many of us only show them hatred. Having someone love on your chubby belly is healing for them. Love them and show them the love they desire, show them gratitude, offer them relief and fill them up with intense nonstop love. They will surprise you with what they offer you in return.

There are two affirmations that we encourage our clients to say on a daily basis:

1. I love myself the same as God love me.
2. I love every inch of my body exactly as it is right now.

If you truly integrate these sayings into your life to the point that you believe it and feel passionate about this belief, you will see a miracle take place in your life. You will wake up feeling enthusiastic about the day ahead, because you will be filled with gratitude for every moment of your life.

Boundaries

So what are healthy boundaries? When we have a firm sense of who we are and what we deserve it is then possible to draw healthy boundaries. But until we begin taking care of ourselves, it is near impossible to set healthy boundaries. Learning to love ourselves comes with change, which comes with resistance. So boundaries will enforce this self-love as you put your needs first in such a way you are more capable of reacting in your best mindset. Give yourself permission to take care of yourself.

1. Love yourself, know who you are, respect yourself and always practice self-care.
   a. Know who you are, what you want and where you're going to truly step out of the need to be perfect for others and set boundaries, we must take the time to get to know ourselves.
   b. Affirmations: to replace faulty core beliefs we must begin changing our self-talk with positive affirmations. Our thoughts become our words and our words become our actions. Our thoughts are like poison to the system, but they can become life to the body when we feed ourselves loving thoughts.
   c. Brainstorm ideas how to better take care of yourself and how to practice daily self-care. Quite often these practices turn into our passions and become who we are.

2. There are healthy physical and healthy emotional boundaries. "People worry that they will hurt or upset people by setting limits or boundaries. For many, love and approval are tied to pleasing others, and setting limits means you are taking a risk that you will not be loved or accepted" – Chad Buck. So how do we create boundaries? And how will they help you?
   a. **Emotions and Limits:** Resentment comes from being taken advantage of or feeling uncomfortable comes from a boundary being crossed. So pay attention to your emotions and give yourself permission to set a boundary when someone's actions create feelings that are less than pleasant.
   b. **Say NO or YES:** The most basic way to establish a boundary is to say no to anything you cannot handle. Sometime we need to be specific and direct with our communication while other times we can be vague and the message still gets across. Sometimes we need a victim protection order (VPO) to set limits. Know what is best for you and follow through by saying NO.
   c. **Respectful yourself:** Give yourself permission to set healthy boundaries. Release the fear of upsetting the other person. Remember you deserve to have boundaries!
   d. **Conscious Creator:** Create your results by following through with your boundaries. Setting a boundary and then allowing others to break them will never align you with your desired result.
   e. **Lifestyle:** Your past does not equal your future, but your past plays a role – this means you have trained others how to treat you. You have reacted in the past to the demands of others and over time they have learned they can use you. Stopping

this pattern will be frustrating, but very rewarding! Start small and progress, always be realistic to set yourself up for success.

f. **Self-Care:** When you give yourself permission to put your own needs first, you can more easily set and stick to your boundaries. It also puts you in a more patient mind frame where you can experience more energy and perspective. Sometimes service will help you to feel love in return better than anything else!

g. **Ask for help:** There's no shame in asking for help. There are support groups everywhere for everything. This is great for finding an accountability buddy too. Call a life coach, a friend or another safe person you trust to talk with. Make sure you are solution focused in finding healthy boundaries and not problem focused where you're just looking for a "rescuer."

h. **Healthy boundaries:** This means no manipulation and no guilt trips. Many of us find ourselves in co-dependent relationships with our family members. Trying to keep them happy while guilt-tripping them for asking. Simply act in a non-defensive manner and do what is best for you in the beginning.

i. **Personal limits:** This includes self-boundaries, treating yourself with respect is huge. NO MORE: self-criticism, self-blaming, self-sabotage, self-hate… MORE: positive self-talk, positive core beliefs, daily affirmations, meditation and self-love. The next time you catch yourself saying, "I look so fat" stop and make this a boundary.

3. The result of healthy Boundaries:
   a. **You are more self-aware:** You can separate your thoughts from your feelings when you begin to recognize your needs.
   b. **Better friend, partner and parent:** You will respect other people's boundaries better too.
   c. **Take better care of yourself:** You can recharge and give yourself permission to take care of yourself, not to mention having more time for yourself.
   d. **Less Stressed:** Everyone has some level of stress, when you set boundaries you will stop making everyone else's problems your own problems too.
   e. **Better communicator:** You will be able to better express your needs. No need to justify yourself.
   f. **More trusting:** Expressing limits means you are trusting others to handle your emotions, which creates better relationships.
   g. **Less angry:** Without boundaries we give our power to others which can lead to anger or a loss of feeling in control. We allow people to do things that aren't ok which makes us more resentful.
   h. **You end up doing things you actually want to do:** All of a sudden you will notice more energy, more happiness, more drive for life, more joyful relationships and more free time to enjoy your life!
   i. **More understanding:** The compassionate people tend to have the best boundaries. This is because you are also compassionate towards yourself when you have a healthy sense of self-worth which leads to healthy boundaries. You can also help others better to heal themselves too.

4. What are some healthy boundaries that you need to make in your life to better take care of yourself:

a. _____

_____

_____

_____

_____

_____

Validation for this New Thought Process

The brain is constantly seeking to be validation for the existing stories, thus creating change takes daily effort. To fully believe the new core belief and the new story you must find validation in the external world to solidify this new belief/story. The words you feed yourself become your belief system. So what are you currently feeding yourself? Has your self-talk shifted since you began this program? Reevaluate your self-talk and notice any patterns of change. This awareness helps you to see your progress so you continue moving forward.

"What the mind of man can see and believe, he can achieve" – Tony Robbins. The body experiences visualizations as if they are real, the power of the mind can create whatever you desire. Believe in the mind and visualize the event working out perfectly. Reality has to conform to your self-image. The old beliefs are comfortable. Fear is nothing more than imagining a negative outcome of a future event. Use this same power to imagine a positive outcome… What future do I want to create? Creating a new path is like a jungle, but as we journey over and over for a few months the new path becomes the new comfort zone. Obviously, the way we have lived in the past didn't work. Shifting the thought process at first requires work, but over time the new thought process will become the automatic natural response.

Visualization: Close your eyes and view yourself from above. View your lifestyle, your family, your job, your home and everything else you have created in your life. Recognize the choices that created this life and the changes you have made. Reflect upon the new understanding you have formed from your past and how the gift of trials and tribulations have created you into who you are today. Take accountability for those achievements as they are no longer holding you hostage, rather you have found the gift in the trial. See how your life is a reflection of new found beliefs, ones that have the potential to create lasting change. Watch yourself facing adversity in the future with grace and faith in God. See this adversity flawlessly working out. Sense the joy filling your heart with pride and humility in the healing grace of your Father in Heaven. Offer Him your gratitude for this gift of life and all that life offers. Accept the gift of agency in all its glory and in its trials. Accept that agency gives us all the right to choose for ourselves even when that choice may bring heartbreak or pain. It is still an opportunity to grow and progress.

Life is temporary and all we struggle with will one day be removed. Imagine yourself visiting the spirit world and reuniting with our lost loved ones. As you do this you will take all of your thoughts, emotions and memories with you. Therefore, healing in the mind is critical for eternal progression so the reward will be accessible in the next life. Invite true forgiveness to sweep into all areas of your mind. Invite self-forgiveness and love for all mankind as you offer others the opportunity to make mistakes too. Accept agency and the healing benefit of the atonement into all areas of your life. Now offer agency and the healing benefit of the atonement to everyone else regardless of their sins. We tend to hold others up to higher expectations than ones we can achieve ourselves. Choose to release this judgmental expectation and invite Christ into your heart as He loves you the same as He loves your enemies. He desires your success and the success of all others. Offer this same Christ-like love to all others upon this planet – living and dead in the same manner Christ has taught.

The scene now takes a shift. All at once you see the world fall into disarray. Horrible scenes from the book of revelations are taking place all around you; war, earthquakes, plagues and starvation. People are struggling with their humanity and suffering terribly. The great cleansing has begun. Your life looks very different. You are living by the grace of God and based off your own preparations. Safety is contingent upon many balancing factors. You may lose a loved one, you may find yourself suffering terribly or you may be alone and frightened. It is easy to change our lives or our perspectives when life is moderate, but when the harsh realities of devastations fall upon us that are outside of our control, the true test begins. When Christ was tried, beaten and crucified, the true test of His character began. He showed us how to love in the midst of His adversity, not just when times are simple or when the trial is over. The way we behave during the most critical of earth's shifts, during the most trying of times, during the most difficult era – that will be the true test of our characters. To heal and solidify a new perspective will offer all that we may need to survive with grace during the great cleansing.

Death is all around you and you are overwhelmed with trials. Offer all your fears, all your heartache and all your condemnation over to the Lord. Let go of all that is not created by God. Let go of all thoughts, emotions and memories that are not a reflection of His great love for you. Fill yourself up with the reassurance of eternal families; you will be reunited once again. The angels are ever present as they watch over you and they even carry you during your trials. Your testimony is forming and service brings you great relief from your suffering. Focus your eyes upon the kingdom of God, prepare your thoughts of worthiness to enter and build up a city worthy of Christ's presence. Your thoughts are powerful and are shared with the angels and the resurrected beings taking residency in the New Jerusalem. Place complete faith in His will and His plan. As devastations occur all around you, place a song of joy in your heart for the return of our King. Keep yourself worthy, find people to serve, share all that you have as it was given through the loving hands of the Savior. He will provide all that you need to survive if you place your faith in Him and if you live the life He has shown by His example. There is nothing to fear as you see the events taking place are glorious to behold.

Raise your eyes to the sky and see the hand of God preparing this amazing city for all those worthy to enter. Watch as you journey throughout the land, offering all you have to others and finding great joy in your service. See yourself step foot into that glorious city. Witness and observe all the angels, the 12 tribes of Israel, and resurrected beings sharing this glorious city with you. Note that you are sharing thoughts, emotions and energy with all those you pass on the streets and as you are building homes. Now as you walk down the street, see your "enemy" – the one person who brought you the most pain in your life. They have found themselves worthy to also enter into this holy city; a place that allows no evil and radiates the light of Christ. Do you feel as though they are worthy of sharing this street with you? Are you welcoming them? Can you feel love for them? Are your emotions leading you towards being unworthy yourself? No emotions created by the adversary are welcome in this city; therefore, are you still worthy to remain?

Cross the street to your "enemy" and offer him or her a hug. Slowly wrap your arms around them and share forgiveness, love, compassion and God's atonement energy with them. The angels begin to sing and you both begin to dance as tears stream down your face. No justification, no excuses, no blame, simply LOVE. Begin to join in the song of the angels during this embrace and allow your spirit to fill with Christ-like love – Text: Joseph L. Townsend

"The day dawn is breaking, the world is awaking, the clouds of night's darkness are fleeing away. The worldwide commotion, from ocean to ocean, now heralds the time of the beautiful day.
Beautiful day of peace and rest, Bright be thy dawn from east to west. Hail to thine earliest welcome ray, Beautiful, bright, millennial day.
In many a temple the Saints will assemble and labor as saviors of dear ones away. Then happy reunion and sweetest communion we'll have with our friends in the beautiful day.
Beautiful day of peace and rest, Bright be thy dawn from east to west. Hail to thine earliest welcome ray, Beautiful, bright, millennial day.
Still let us be doing, our lessons reviewing, Which God has revealed for our walk in his way; and then, wondrous story, the Lord in his glory will come in his pow'r in the beautiful day.
Beautiful day of peace and rest, Bright be thy dawn from east to west. Hail to thine earliest welcome ray, Beautiful, bright, millennial day.
Then pure and supernal, our friendship eternal, With Jesus we'll live, and his counsels obey until ev'ry nation will join in salvation and worship the Lord of the beautiful day.
Beautiful day of peace and rest, Bright be thy dawn from east to west. Hail to thine earliest welcome ray, Beautiful, bright, millennial day."

You can open your eyes and soak up the love and the healing energy available to you.

Assignments

Energy Work:

1. Test for the most critical energy to release. Be sure the translucent energy is completed before taking the next step and the destructive energies. Be sure the most critical dark energies have also been removed. Pay close attention to removing the most severe dark energies before continuing: the addiction dark, dark dark, chaos, death and revenge, discouragement and suicide, no will to live, fear dark, destructive dark, control dark, deceived dark and sexual dark.
2. Create a healing compound. Use the Compounds and Charts Manual.
3. Test for further needs of your client regarding food. With the changes taking place regarding energy releases, some foods can be reintroduced. Ask the body what it needs to continue healing. Go through a list of healing foods and a list of current intolerances. Use the Compounds and Charts book for references to healing foods.

Homework:

1. Practice a daily visualization of your new consciousness playing into all avenues of your life. Witness God's actions in your life and envision the future with this new Christ-like perspective.
2. Pray daily and practice changing your prayers to resemble a more loving conversation where you are a tool of service for others. Pray for your enemies until you begin to love your enemies as your own brother/sister.
3. Continue all your previous assignments regarding affirmations. Add any affirmations that are necessary to continue progressive thought patterns. (See Appendix page 123)
4. Test for a tapping sequence needed to continue balancing hormones and solidifying the new thought patterns, found in the Appendix.

Self-Sabotage
Step Ten

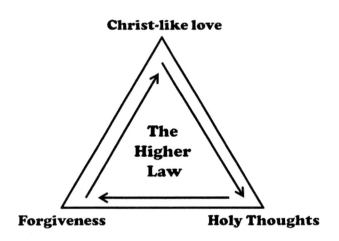

Christ-like love

The
Higher
Law

Forgiveness   **Holy Thoughts**

Clear Your Space

Test your client to see if these steps need to be completed before continuing. These steps are found in the Appendix. Always begin your appointments by checking for "attacks."

1. Begin by clearing the space and removing all dark influences/rebellious spirits
2. Remove Self-Destructive Tools of Dark Influences
3. Remove Mind Subconscious suggestions
4. Remove Intimidation Energy
5. Ask for shields of protection

~~~~~~

The Outward View

In the introduction we emphasize the need for an internal change. Throughout this manual we are working towards creating an internal change, which is primarily geared towards the way in which we view ourselves. We often compare ourselves to others, which leads to self-criticism and fault finding in others. In some cases we will see others excel and become envious of their success and look for ways to put them down to make ourselves feel better. When we look at life as always a competition of who is better than who, we will always lose. There is no race to the finish line.

Recognizing the joy we have in the success of close family members can be a good place to begin looking outwards. Remembering that we are all brothers and sisters upon this earth will help us view others in a more loving nature. If we look at life as an opportunity to mature with our fellow brothers and sisters who we desperately desire to assist, then we are set on a successful course.

In the book, "Healing from Above," Alexandria and Calvin provided some insightful words that teach about shifting our self-critical perspective to focus upon our Savior.

"When the self-sabotage energies take over, one tends to look inward, focusing primarily upon their own faults and flaws and shortcomings. **One misses the opportunities to be uplifted by looking outward.** When looking inward becomes so overwhelming, the energy radiating from you is negative and others stray from your presence. It bounces and drags others down which in turn drags you further down, it's a vicious cycle which is ironic because the person suffering feels such guilt for dragging others down that they sink deeper and deeper… Choosing to look outward and no longer focus upon oneself must be one of the latter steps in your process. Shift the perspective from self-critical to self-love regardless of imperfections. And **focusing upon the savior, <u>this focus corrects the impulse to be self-critical,</u> because you begin seeing yourself and others as Christ sees them, slowly becoming more like Christ every day**." – Healing From Above: Conversations with Angels Book One by Alexandria and Calvin

This falls in line with the verse spoken by Christ, "For whosoever will save his life shall lose it: but whosoever will lose his life for my sake, the same shall save it" – Luke 9: 24 (KJV). These words may seem simple and easy to apply to life; however, pride and selfishness often creep into our daily lives. The apostle Paul teaches us in Galatians 5: 22-23 that the "fruit of the spirit is love, joy, peace, longsuffering, gentleness, goodness, faith, meekness, temperance." (KJV) These are the type of attributes that we are working towards as we overcome self-sabotage. These are the type of strengths that come with those that possess an outward view in life. When we "lose" our life, we are handing it over to Christ. We are not searching for ways in which we can rise above other; rather, we are searching for ways in which we can serve others.

Consider who might need your help today. Practice self-care in the form of service today. My favorite service project is done with my children; we gather food from around the house that is packaged up and we fill multiple grocery bags. Then we include a book- typically a self-help book or scriptures or a spiritual book along with a note of affirmation words. Most times it says "God Loves You" Then we put the bags in the car waiting for the right moment. As we are driving together throughout the week, there is always an opportunity where a homeless man or woman is on the street corner. I take the time to park the car and offer them the prepared bag along with a hug and a few kind words of love. The touch and loving words is crucial in this offering of service. Remember your brothers and sisters that are less fortunate than you.

Ask yourself, "What is God's will for me today?" and take the time to hear the answer. Quite often we ask, but quickly go about our day unwilling to wait for the answer. Take the time today to wait and listen for His answer. Then follow through and take the action steps!

The Higher Law

The higher law of Moses comes with greater responsibilities that one must live up to in order to dwell in the presence of God. It must come through the proper authority; therefore, I am not teaching the higher law at this time, I am simply explaining how to prepare to live the higher law. We must also know what it means to live the higher law in our worldly understanding.

Stating it simply, it takes place within your thoughts, emotions and energy fields. Complete healing is not attained, nor bought; but it is lived every day. You cannot look upon the past with ill feelings. This is not accomplished without effort. Drawing upon the energy of the Lord is a simple task of asking and receiving. He shall share His strength and understanding and even His level with you at any given moment. This will elevate your frequencies and vibrations to be aligned with the Savior, not just your own desires.

We then move a step further by drawing upon the powers of heaven and allowing the clouds to part and shine down their heavenly rays upon your mind. Communicate with your spirit and ask for your spirit to open its secret compartments upon your mind for further knowledge of God's plan and purpose. Ask for further light and knowledge at the will of God, but be open enough to receive. Allow your own understanding to be increased as you humble yourself to the Lord's divinity. Focus your thoughts on humility, teachability, gentleness, compassion and spirituality. Your spirit has the power to move a mountain, this is true, but your mind does not. It is not comprehensive unto the physics and laws of man, neither is it possible to walk on water…. Or is it? Is there a purpose at this time or would it be for greed and fortune, fame or recognition. If the heart is centered upon the will of God and not your own and if the heart is softened unto the ways of God while turning away from the natural man, you shall see a shift naturally occur. This shift takes years of patience as it brings a testimony centered in Christ and His gospel. When you allow your mind to open its hidden compartments or secret chakra, your spirit can bear witness unto the power of His work and glory. I know it sounds simple and yet it is not. This shift will open your eyes and you will see your past through different eyes. Your emotions will respond differently and you will feel compassion further while expanding your limitations less.

Move forward with a leap, a skip, a twirl and dance while singing praises unto Him for He possesses the most amazing miracle of life, joy and utter bliss. You've felt it in your heart and you have seen it change your perspective into a miracle of love. Prayer for your enemies is just the first step as there are many steps with each first step. **Do not stop moving your feet and you will hear the song.** Your heart is changing and the view within your mind's eyes will be shared with many others as you learn how to form words for the things you can understand and see. Your perspective is limited when you place time constraints upon your perspective. When you remove the limitations, it opens up into a new understanding as a simple angle is replaced with one you didn't know existed. Frequently, visit your previous lessons as they will continue to teach you new guidance as your perspective continues to shift.

How do you fully forgive? How do you live the higher law? How does one fly? Well, your spirit does not fly by focusing on flying, because the mind restricts the flight. But **when you focus on the Savior and heaven's gates you will find yourself soaring through the sky**. This is the exact same concept in the higher law. Become forgiving in your heart so naturally that you never reach a level of intensity in the first place. Live as the Savior lived... I want to add something here. If you try to have perfect thoughts, perfect lives and you aspire to live the higher law; it is easier to pluck a honeybee from the inside of a black olive under the filthy river where the current is pulling you in the opposite direction. This does not mean to give up and run in the other direction. This does not mean to make excuses for the inability to reach the impossible expectations and simply remain in the filthy waters too burdened to proceed.

Father has laid out a plan. He has given us steps. Once you have mastered the Ten Commandments, go to the next step. Begin the law of chastity, the word of wisdom and find your testimony. You do not simply create a peaceful, churchgoer out of thin air; you work at it every day until it becomes WHO you are. Once these steps are mastered and you seek enjoyment out of obedience and service, then you move on and begin perfecting yourself. Service is the single most effective way to offer Christ-like love. You don't do this alone or without effort. You find love internally and share it externally. You invite the light of Christ to radiate from your being, because it is who you are and it comes naturally from within. Loving yourself needs to be mastered prior to this step, because this takes it to the next level. Seeing your body and existence as a divine grand gesture of love comes after learning to love the imperfections that the world places upon you.

Your thoughts do begin at the beginning. When a lifetime of faulty thoughts has escalated to unreasonable assumptions and negative outlooks, this is far from the time to aspire to the higher law. But when you have gained that testimony from obedience, then you are ready for the next step. Obedience in the thought processes seems to reflect upon your ability to love fully and forgive fully. When forgiveness ceases to be difficult, you know you have arrived. When your thoughts naturally play into a healing dynamic of love for all mankind, one of equality for even the highest and lowest of spirits, you know you have arrived. Most people who are living the higher law do not boast nor do they reach a point of simply stating, "I'm done progressing." They continue improving, they seek constant growth. Complacency is not a word they know. They are ever growing, even when they are seen as perfect. This is what makes them worthy in God's eyes, because they are not seeking their own desires, but that of God's. Effortless work is bound by the enemy. However, the work of the Lord is ever seeking improvement and growth, this makes His plan infinite with loving possibilities. To seek these steps are still yet just a baby step in the grand overall picture.

The Higher Law. Moses brought forth more commandments than the 10 we have in the scriptures. Although these commandments have been lost, this is not an excuse to live a worldly life and disregard the higher law. The top 10 are really the most simple and basic. When you are ready to go above and beyond you'll be thirsty for the next step. This step is laced in the scriptures with the manner Christ lived His life. We know He is perfect, but many times we simply stop pushing ourselves and become complacent with mediocrity.

The amount of energy that our spirit, mind and bodies can contain within is absolutely incredible. With this in mind, we need to consider the amount of negative energy that is being stored as well. There is far too much to release some energies here and there. Our goal for our clients is to be able to release all of their negative energy and live a Christ-like life so that the negative influences will be minimalized. A full release is something that needs to come from the heart and involves the atonement. Remember that Christ is the one that heals!

Veil Free Will Conversion

The energies that we hold within us were originally created by God. With this in mind, we can assume that the energies were originally created as a positive energy. We can also assume that the energy has at least a small form of intelligence that will always desire to become the most positive form of energy it possibly can. We are the ones that take these positive forms of energy and restrict their free will, thus converting them into a negative energy.

Throughout life we experience a wide range of emotions. We can view the same event either in a positive or negative manner. When we hold onto an experience that we view as negative we trap the emotions associated with that experience. "Trapping" them is the key term here. After the event has past, if we don't take the time to consciously let the negative emotions go, we end up storing them. We may hope to forget them or we may continue to trap them in hopes to find validation for those feelings. Meanwhile, the emotions continue to wreak havoc within the body long past the time the event occurred. With a conscious effort, we can let all of our past emotions free.

Heavenly Father has offered us a veil of forgetfulness. This veil is holy and righteous, it is not meant to be tampered with. However, Lucifer has created an opposite to all of God's righteous creations. Our spirits know our divinity and, therefore, when this sin is against the higher law, we will create a veil to hide from God. Similar to when Adam and Eve were in the Garden of Eden; God came to visit and they hid in shame due to their nakedness. The adversary told them to hide or Father would see. These veil energies are very similar. When we sin in our thoughts or against the higher law or we feel ashamed of ourselves, even if nobody else knew, we feel the need to hide our sin from God. So we create a veil, much like a curtain, to hide our sins. Ironically, this veil doesn't keep God from seeing us in our vulnerable state, but He does respect our privacy. This veil may be created by you, but you were influenced by the rebellion. This release can be done one by one or all together based on the needs of your client. This is a free will conversion of all veils and all veil energies by showing the energy our love, setting it free and inviting it to choose whether it would like to remain as a negative energy or to be converted into a positive energy. It's always important to incorporate the atonement into a release for complete healing and to assist in creating lasting change in the behavior or thought process that created the energy originally. Test if this is best for your client before proceeding.

Energy work: "I bring to light all veil energies, energetic connections, cords, the words, thoughts, memories, loops, veils, excess, toxicity and all other components that are associated with the veil energies.

I ask for God to shine the light of truth upon all energy within me. I ask this light to organize this energy and the creations of this energy into compartments. These compartments will divide that which leads me towards God and that which leads me away from God. While doing this release we will now focus upon the energies that lead me away from God.

I offer these energies my love as they have been part of me and have taught me many things. I know that I have to experience the bad in order to learn the good. I am ready to let go of my past, since the past is not who I am and the negativity no longer serves me. I choose to shift my perspective to a more loving and thankful approach to challenging situations. I will look for opportunities to grow and expand my talents, rather than hiding them under a bushel.

I offer all of the veil energies their free will. I no longer desire to hold onto them and I let them go. I allow them the choice to depart from spirit, mind, body and energy fields or if they would like to remain as a positive energy within me and assist me in the healing process, they may do so. I remind this energy of its original creation and the purpose for which God created it. I also let go of all connections to the veil energies. I specifically let go of the energetic connections and the cords. I send my love into the connections and cords and invite them convert into positive forms of energy. I also send my love into all those who I have these connections with and I apologize to them for the harm I have caused them. I also apologize to my spirit for storing this negativity within and I commit to living a life filled with love towards myself and others, so that I no longer hold onto negative emotions.

I shine the light of truth upon all of the words, thoughts and memories. I send my love and understanding into each word, thought and memory. I invite each word, thought and memory to allow a shift in their perspective and to be converted into positive, life affirming words, thoughts and memories that will build my confidence and strengthen my spirit, mind and body. I let go of all connection to them and allow them their free will. I invite them to be distributed throughout my body in any location that they desire. I place my trust in these new words, thoughts and memories and thank them for the light and understanding they offer to me.

I have created all these veils to hide my shame from God. I now send my love into these veils and I offer them free will. I thank these energies for being part of me and helping me to learn. I let them go, along with all attachments to them. I remind the energies within the veils of their original creation and the purpose for which God created them.

I send my love into all remaining veil energy components within my spirit, mind, body and energy fields and I offer them free will. I thank these energies for being part of me and helping me to learn. I let them go, along with all attachments and I invite them to be converted into positive forms of energy. I remind the energies of their original creation and the purpose for which God created them. I invite my mind to form new loops that are congruent with the new words, thoughts and memories. I invite vibrations from the sun to combine with my vibrations. I invite the raised vibrations to breathe life into the circuits in my mind; continuously feeding a new thought process/energy that will lead towards the higher understanding of Father in Heaven.

I thank the earth for her endless service in my behalf. I invite the earth to bless me with her healing energies for the purpose of breaking down the toxicity within me that was created by the negative energies. I also ask her to bless me with her healing energies for the purpose of breaking down the excess that was formed to store the energies and to heal the damage caused by the energies.

I ask that my spirit, mind and body recognize the changes that have taken place and adjust accordingly. I invite my body to realign my organs, bones, tissue and all other parts of my body to their proper location, now that the veil energies have been removed.

Lastly, I recognize the mistakes I made that formed this energy. I thank my Lord and Savior, Jesus Christ for the atonement and I invite my Father in Heaven and my Savior into my heart and I allow them to see me fully and completely. I accept the life of Jesus Christ and His blood that was shed for me. I invite and accept the atonement energy into my spirit, mind and body. I invite God to cleanse me, purify me and make me clean – as white as snow, as I bury my past and renew myself through the atonement. I choose to commit to change and I commit to live my life in accordance with the commandments of God. I dedicate my life to my Lord and Savior, Jesus Christ, and I accept His name. I invite the Holy Spirit into my life. I offer unconditional love to my Creator; and I offer unconditional love to all my brothers and sisters - living and dead."

~~~~~~

Self-Sabotage Mountain

Even when we take significant steps to clear out the baggage in our minds, there is still a mountain of memories that seem to haunt us. They affect self-talk, dreams, sleeping habits, body shape, and relationships. They just seem to rear their ugly little heads every time we are making any progress in life, creating the perfect self-sabotage. This can feel discouraging, as if the past is disabling any hopes for recovery.

I'll share a personal story about this. I experienced a significant amount of trials for my age, maybe to the extreme. I finally remarried in 2016, but even with all my personal development work and energy work, I have still struggled with memories. I had forgiven and been able to feel love for others, but I have struggled with the negativity surrounding these events as if there was another form of control being exercised against me on occasion. I have done all the possible energy work on myself and I know it is an ongoing opportunity, but I still would sabotage my own progress with self-doubt or fears from my past. The difficulty of moving on after divorce is hard enough without adding a level of disconnection. So what else can we do to fully heal? How can we share a room with someone who created terrible distress in our lives and feel only peace for them? We know healing is through faith in God and takes time. It is not time that passes the pain, time is only a measurement of opportunities to heal. Are you taking the appropriate steps every day to naturally create results you want AND do you believe you deserve those results?

So here's what we found when we dove into the cause of my self-sabotage pattern; there was a MOUNTAIN of repressed memories. A whole mountain! Not a tiny little hill either, but a mountain as big and intense of a climb as Everest!

Let's call this a self-sabotage mountain of repressed memories. I like to think of repressed memories as the body's way of protecting you from serious traumatic memories, but if they keep negatively affecting you, something must be done. Let's do a visualization once again to deal with this mountain. Have you noticed how many visualizations we do? It's amazing how the mind has such power to create the reality you desire or to change your reality simply due to intentions. You might have started realizing that your thoughts have significant power which means negative thoughts are just as powerful.

Energy work: Remove the contracted rebellious spirit to this mountain and the energy that created it.

1. "I bring to light the rebellious spirit and the cords/chains and the contract. I command this contract be washed in the living waters. I detach all chains/cords, I cut these cords with the living sword, I release the cords and I remove the cords. I ask the hounds to chew off the remaining chains. I offer you 3 choices – repent and become and angel in training, depart or you will be cast out." (Visualize these steps and follow through if you must remove the rebellious spirit. Take your time on these steps.)
2. I bring to light the frequencies and vibrations of all energy that created this mountain in the spirit, mind, body and energy fields. I command all this energy into a portal. I detach the cords, I cut those cords with the healing sword, I release the cords and I remove the cords. I seal the portal at all openings in the name of Jesus Christ, never to be reopened.

Visualization: Close your eyes and imagine you are sitting in your home; this is a million dollar mansion, your dream home. This mansion was gifted to you by a wealthy mentor. When you moved in, this home was immaculate and in perfect condition. This home was given to you; you can destroy it, manage it, or improve it. The house is beautiful on the outside and presentable to the neighbors, you fit right in.

After settling in and living in this mansion for many years, this mansion looks very different on the inside as it was very difficult to maintain. Over the years your home has slowly become a hoarder's house. You don't know exactly how it happened, just slowly over time stuff began to pile up. There is trash piled to the ceiling in every room, all the bedrooms are barricaded with stuff you don't need or use. Dishes overflow onto the floor, the bathrooms aren't functioning, and furniture is torn up and uncomfortable as they are covered in fecal matter from the excess of pets you rescued. You cannot even climb into bed to receive rest because there is so much "stuff" blocking the way, you aren't even sure you could find the bed if you tried. The amount of work to clean up is overwhelming and leaves you feeling drained and defeated.

You have one tiny spot that is clean where you spend most of your time and that is in front of the windows facing the street. You find a great deal of comfort and peace in this small space, but the amount of work ahead is overwhelming and it feels easier to stuff it all away into another room and quickly shut the door… Like you have been doing for many years. Unfortunately, it's starting to spill out of those rooms and it is now affecting your ability to breathe clean air, your ability to relax or receive rest. You are embarrassed to have anyone over so you keep everyone out of your home for fear of them seeing what's inside. You no longer want to continue living this way.

Imagine walking outside. Allow the fresh air to brush your face and invite in the healing elements of the sunlight into your body. Now kneel down and pray. Ask God for help. Remember you are as a little child who needs help at times and this happens to be bigger than you are. Recognize you just can't do this alone. Instantly a bright light appears as Christ walks towards you. He waits patiently until you are ready to hand over this huge burden and let go of the result; the stress, the shame, and the embarrassment. Invite Him to fully see you knowing He will never judge you as He loves you completely with a love that requires nothing in exchange. Invite God into your home and trust in Him with everything that is hidden inside. Once you are ready we will move on (pause for confirmation to proceed).

As you are kneeling, look back at your home and see the Savior walking inside. He goes from room to room opening windows and observing your living conditions. All at once a bright light radiates from the windows. The roof becomes like crystal glass as light comes in freely and exits freely. The walls begin to move and shift as the spirit within the wood is experiencing joy in its creation. The creation of this home is being magnified into a potential you had never known possible. The walls seem to sing, the air is rejoicing, the items within are coming to life in such a way that brings great joy. The longer Christ is inside the more your home seems to glow with light and love. All at once the angels begin to sing and surround your lovely home singing praises unto God. Light comes down from the heavens and your home begins to pour forth love and light and healing energy. This energy seems to have a mission and a spirit itself. You watch this light ray as it travels throughout your entire home, within the walls and even along the external bricks. This light is alive and radiates the light of the atonement as it continues to travel throughout the entire creation of your home and even into every particle of its existence. Nothing is forgotten. Your home becomes glorious and magnificent to behold. You feel a desire to go back inside as it now brings you great joy.

When you walk inside, you see something you have never seen before. Exponential value, cleanliness, order, and you begin feeling proud of this home of yours. You walk from room to room and see the filth has been made clean. What was broken is now working. The excess of stuff has been organized into piles. Each one is labeled. Donate, share, keep, fix, recycle, trash. You are rather curious of this organization system. Christ explains to you: the "donation" items represent all that was once usable and necessary, but no longer needed; stuff you need to let go. The "share" items represent items you can use to uplift others, to share little by little with those who cross your path to improve their lives. The "keep" items represent personal items that need to remain because it offers comfort, safety and happiness. These items can be visible to guests or family and can also become a part of your wardrobe to represent your personality. The "fix" items represent items remaining that are broken and needing extra special attention, something valuable that can become beautiful again with a little creativity. These items are to remind you of the value of hard work and how sometimes the past leaves scars, but can be reinvented into something else more useful than before. The "recycle" items represent what was highly useful, but ready to become converted into another item with a complete transformation. The "trash" pile represents items that no longer serve anyone, items that need to be removed as they only bring a remembrance of filth.

The angels quickly tend to these piles and remove that which is ready to be removed. The trash and recycle pile is removed completely. The donation items are removed and taken to others who are currently in the place you once were. The share and keep items are nicely organized within your home but the "keep" items are put away. The "fix" items remain as Christ places them gently in a row and steps back to stand by your side. He asks you if you would like some assistance creating a work of art. You accept and together you tackle each item, one by one. You watch as His hands seem to glide over the workings and components as if He had a deep respect and love for the spirit within. You ask Him to lead, while working together as a team. You find great joy in participating in this grand gesture of service and productivity. Time seems to pass quickly and all the items that were once broken are instead recreated into beautiful workings of art. As you look at each one, they are far more beautiful than before, they have more useful purposes and they each seem to encompass love as they represent hard work, a second chance and a new creation. Each one is stronger than before.

Christ asks you if you would like to see the improvements. You agree and He walks with you from room to room. The space is clean, organized and livable. The family room has a sofa to rest upon and socialize with friends. Your bedroom has a magnificent canopy bed with draping's made of a shimmery glowing fabric that seems to dance with the wind coming in from the windows. You have a library/office filled wall to wall with books to expand your mind. The kitchen is full of nutritious food that is welcome and offers strength and vitality. The water is beaming with the joy of its creation as it is alive. The items within your home are useful, they bring you joy and you see how each have a function created perfectly. **This home is designed to sustain life.** It is designed to protect you from the storms of life. It is open for many to enter in and find loving safety within. Everything about your home now breathes life and energy. The roof is permanently made of crystal glass facing upwards as it is open to the heavens for a source of energy, strength and light.

You desire to share this home with others. You begin to imagine how you want your spouse, kids and friends to share in the beauty of this home. You even desire to find ways to serve others with this home as it is a gift, one that you finally are ready to share with others. You feel a deep level of respect for your home and you desire to change the ways you treat your home. You learned how you cared for this home in the past brought suffering and therefore with this fresh start, you desire to keep your home to clean. You commit to change so you may experience a better result in the future as maintenance requires daily effort.

Christ offers you a hug and says His goodbyes. You thank Him for offering you everything He has; His time, talents, and love. He kisses your forehead and departs into a ray of bright light. Energy, love and excitement fill your heart as you find great joy in the value of your home. What a treasure to be gifted such an amazing creation to house your spirit. One that is like unto a temple as it is worthy of reverence, respect, kindness, patience, forgiveness, order, and the light of the atonement. You commit to maintaining this beautiful home and even improving it every day in the ways Christ showed you through His loving example.

Imagine inviting all the healing light that traveled through your home into your body, mind and spirit and watch as it journeys into every crevice, avenue and location; offering healing light freely. This light can be experienced anytime you so choose. Then invite and absorb into your body compassion, tolerance, love and peace to freely flow as a fountain of living energy continuously flowing throughout your being.

Open your eyes and speak some kind, loving words of affirmations to yourself.

~~~~~~

Assignments

Energy work:

1. Test for the energy that created the self-sabotage mountain and do this release IF it's still remaining.
2. Retest to see what remaining dark energies your client still has. The living energies will remain as they are a conscious lifestyle; meaning they are the experiences/trials currently being lived. These may need to be released more than once as agency remains.
3. Continue releasing trauma energies or sensory energies or addictive energies or sexual energies if any remain. The sensory energies include healing the RNA and the DNA as does the physical trauma so the body may still need these steps performed.

Homework:

1. Continue daily self-care.
2. Practice your new boundaries daily.
3. Meditate daily.
4. Test for additional affirmations needed to reform healthier thought processes.
5. Visualize this healing light daily and visualize your life's circumstances being resolved.
6. Do a service project.
7. Focus on reinforcing your positive self-talk all day every day.

Self-Sabotage

Step Eleven

Clear Your Space

Test your client to see if these steps need to be completed before continuing. These steps are found in the Appendix. Always begin your appointments by checking for "attacks."

1. Begin by clearing the space and removing all dark influences/rebellious spirits
2. Remove Self-Destructive Tools of Dark Influences
3. Remove Mind Subconscious suggestions
4. Remove Intimidation Energy
5. Ask for shields of protection

~~~~~~

Full Release of Negative Energy

A few things to recognize with a full release:

1. Not everyone will initially be ready for this. A full release is appropriate for those at a level 7 and above. Individuals with a frail body may have difficulty with this. Muscle test to see if this is safe for the client. If a client is unable to do a full release, they may still be able to release several energies at once. For instance, releasing all of the veil energies can be done for those at a level 6.
2. Live energies (energies that are currently being lived/experienced) are likely to return as the person re-engages the situation that involves these energies.
3. The curses associated with the dark energies might remain. The dark energies are also alive, so it is best to release live energies individually, especially the dark energies; however each person's success is based upon their faith.
4. This is fantastic maintenance, but the spirit, mind, and body has learn the "how to" steps prior to this release. The assignments cannot be skipped if this is to be successful.

The purpose of doing a full release is to prepare to live the higher law which allows no negative energy, emotions or thoughts that are not created by God; to reside within your spirit, mind or body. Step into your power and speak this release with confidence and decisiveness. You can do this by proxy and interactively so as you speak, ask your client to follow along as if everything you say takes place within their mind as well.

Energy work: Lie down, relax your body, close your eyes and visualize Godly light entering into your body. This light is living and glorious as it invites healing and loving energy to flow through your body. Watch it come in from the atmosphere and all around into every avenue of your body. Focus on the divinity of your body, this grand creation of God's handiwork. Allow the light of Christ to shine from within you brighter and brighter until your light is shining throughout the entire universe. Simultaneously, visualize negative energy leaving your body; watch it flow out your hands, toes and all other areas of your being. Choose to reject, release and remove all negative energy influenced by the rebellion. Place faith within your own ability to heal and the ability within your spirit. Have faith in God and remember you are loved.

"I bring to light all frequencies and vibrations of all energy within me. All creations of God within my body, mind and spirit. I bring to light all creations of the rebellion within my body, mind and spirit. I bring to light all types of influences and their effect upon my body.

I choose to see all influences in their true form as I ask God to shine His light upon my spirit, mind and body to reveal the true origin of all emotions and memories within me.

In the name of Jesus Christ I command all rebellious spirits to depart from all cords, all attachments, from anything and everything that is connected to me or is within me or my space. I seal any and all portals in any of these spaces and command them to never be reopened. I strengthen my shields as they are connected to my spirit, they are a part of me and they protect my free will and my ability to make healthy clean choices for myself.

I cleanse all attachments as I shine the light of the atonement into all cords and connections. I choose to convert them into loving opportunities for forgiveness and healing love. I release all connections, cords or attachments that no longer serve me.

I detach all negative connections I have with anybody else in relation to any and all negative energy within me at this time. I separate myself from these connections, offering myself the space and freedom to heal in my own time and in my own ways. I place a wall between me and anyone else sharing any of these energies and this wall will offer Christ-like love to anyone attempting to recreate these connections. I detach any and all negative cords attached to me, attached to others and these negative energies and I untie all cords that can be untied. I send loving energy, forgiveness and understanding into these negative cords to convert them with the healing power of the atonement. I cut any remaining negative cords with the sword of love and I release all these cords and I remove all these cords.

I neutralize and defuse all frequencies and vibrations of all dark energies, traumas and all other negative energies created by the rebellion or influenced by the rebellion. that are in my spirit, mind, body, and energy fields. I command this energy to depart from my body and out of existence. I detach all cords, I cut those cords with the revolving sword and I release and remove those cords.

I bring to light all rebellious spirits and their contracts connected to me. I command the contracts to be washed in the living waters or burned with the light of Christ. I detach the

98

cords/chains to the rebellious spirits, I cut these cords with the sword of the rebellion and I ask the hounds to chew off any remaining chains. I release and remove the chains/cords. You are no longer welcome, the energy has been removed, and therefore, you must leave. I say unto you repent and become an angel in training. Remember your purpose, your life and your agency. If you choose not to repent then you are free to leave, but if you choose to remain and attack – then in the name of Jesus Christ I command the remaining rebellious spirits to depart immediately! I seal all portals in the appropriate manner, which seals all openings completely and permanently. I command all portals to be cast out of creation.

I strengthen my shields and ask for the love of God to lace through my shields. I also ask for the light rod to God to lace throughout my exterior shield for the purpose of protection against destructive energies.

I allow all negative energy to flow out of my body; out of my center being, through my arms or legs and out my toes or fingers. I release all this negative energy as it no longer has a place within me. (*Imagine seeing all the negativity flow out.*) Any remaining energy I offer the gift of agency; to forgive and convert through the healing power of the atonement into positive flowing life affirming energy.

I recognize all damage that has occurred to my body. I also recognize how this body has worked so hard to survive and protect me. I awaken all burned out senses and switches. I choose to untie all knotted or blocked flows of energy. I open my chakras to God to heal the damage that has occurred due to the difficulty and complications of life.

I invite into my body, mind and spirit the light of the atonement as forgiveness is the greatest gift I can offer myself and others. Agency offers freedom; I choose to offer agency to others as it was gifted to me freely. I also choose to allow others to be imperfect as I forgive their infractions upon me; I too pray they forgive my infractions upon them. I choose to see my imperfections in a space of safety where I need no barriers, because I am loved exactly as I am right now by God. I invite into my space, my mind, my spirit and my body; peace and love, self-acceptance, self-worth and God's love. I invite all love and acceptance into my space and into my body. I invite in the healing light of love for my brothers and sisters as I choose to honor the gift of agency and the gift of this life. I choose to see all others upon this planet, as children of God with the same divinity as I possess.

I invite and absorb into my meridian a continuous fountain of flowing healthy energy: spiritual emotions, positive emotions, love and strength of spirit animals, nutrients, herbs, healthy bacteria, oils within the earth and atmosphere, food and ionized water. I also invite and absorb into my meridian elements of the earth, light or sound energy waves and hormones. I invite all this healing energy to be distributed throughout my body to replace any depletion and break down all the excess tissue, all toxins, all infections and to heal all illness in all areas that need assistance in healing. I recognize that my body is lovingly taking care of me and lovingly protecting me. I invite these elements to concentrate or merge or combine in their respective ways for the healing of this body so it may function in the manner in which my loving Heavenly Father created my body to function.

I allow myself a safe space to move forward and to move on in my progression in this life. No longer living in the past, no longer living in the future, but living mindfully in the present, being free to experience all that Father has to offer, ready and willing to invite in more experiences. As more situations are presented to me and more emotions are experienced and events are brought into my life, I acknowledge my feelings. I acknowledge my emotions, but I no longer hold onto them. I do not need to store negative energy. I release all negative energy as it comes towards me, as I experience it. I do not store it. I let it go right back out my body as I choose to continuously only invite in good to stay. I only wish to have positive loving thoughts, because I love myself. I love my life and I am so grateful for this opportunity to be alive that I choose to feed myself life affirming words and thoughts. I choose a perspective least obscured by imperfections or ill worded opinions of others. I do not need other people's acceptance or approval as I love myself. If someone else uses harsh words towards me, I do not store these words. I do not ignore these words either, instead I offer so much love and so much positivity that I in turn lift others and bring them the love of my Father in Heaven.

I am ready to progress in my existence. I am aware now of the emotions and energies created by God and I am aware of the emotions and energies influenced by the rebellion. I no longer wish to wear a mask and sink into self-sabotage when I know my true purpose in life. I exist due to a loving God who desires I grow and progress in life. He knows I will stumble. He knows I am imperfect. I am like a little child learning, growing, and changing. God forgives me for my past as He sees my potential. I too forgive myself for my past. I forgive others for mistakes they have made in the past. I forgive myself and others for mistakes we will surely make in the future. It's ok to be human as I am designed for change and progression. In this same regard I choose to strive to become more like my Savior Jesus Christ. He is my brother who has given me an example of who I wish to be. He is my mentor, my brother and my friend. I value His life, His sacrifice and His existence. I know I deserve His love. I deserve the gift of His atonement.

This body was created with love in the image of God. My Heavenly Parents love me enough to craft an entire planet for me. My Heavenly Parents love me as much as they love my enemies. I choose to pray for my enemies and convert all my feelings into love for all others regardless of the choices they make. This is how my loving Savior has taught me to love. I choose to see myself as a divine creation of my Heavenly Parents. My body is a trusted item that is capable of far more than I have been aware in the past, but I am starting to see my true worth. I am opening my eyes to my value in the manner God sees me. I cannot fully love in the manner God loves, but I am learning. I choose to set myself up for success and expand my comfort zone into a more Godly understanding of my divinity. I ask God to open my eyes and show me the true nature of my existence. I open my mind to a new understanding of my divine nature. My body is a precious commodity; every emotion, every experience, every sensation is holy. I am blessed to view myself from a space of pure honesty given to me through the understanding only God can offer. I no longer choose to believe the false teachings of the adversary or the rebellion. All energy that is Godly is invited into my space, but any energy that is created by the rebellion, I choose to reject. My spirit, mind and body deserve clean thoughts, clean actions, clean memories and clean relationships. As a spirit child of God I know my purpose and I know my potential. As a mortal with a body of flesh and blood, it is my job to keep holding onto the straight and narrow path towards my Lord and Savior Jesus Christ, the path towards eternal life.

When I slip, I can quickly get back upon my feet, because I know I am forgiven. The hardest person to forgive is myself. I apologize to my spirit, I apologize to my Father in Heaven and I apologize to all those I have harmed. I forgive all my brothers and sisters. I know their worth is just as valuable as my own, I know Father in Heaven desires their success as well as my own. I forgive myself because there is no need to hold onto my past. My past is just a stumbling block to teach me how to walk forward differently than I planned while trusting in God. I know my past is forgivable. I choose to move forward with a more complete understanding of the purpose of life and how these experiences are for my own good. I accept Heavenly Father's forgiveness as I see He understands on a level much higher than my own. He sees me as a little child who is precious beyond words. He desires I keep trying, He wants me to progress, He wants me to learn from my mistakes, He wants me to see the magnificent individual He sees in me.

I know this gift of agency can be heartbreaking at times, but I still choose God's plan. I know other people can choose evil and that evil can hurt me or my family, but I still choose God's plan. Sometimes it's hard to "not know" the outcome or cause of so much suffering, but I choose to trust God as He knows the larger picture and I choose His plan. God can see my entire existence and He knows what's best for me. I will trust in Him with my future, my past and every second of my life. True healing, true peace and true happiness comes through God and His plan of salvation. Although it may be hard at times, I choose to see the gift in my trials so I may learn how to grow.

My body, my mind and my spirit are each precious in their own respect. From now on, I will cherish this gift that's limited to this short time I have on earth. I am overwhelmed with gratitude for the opportunity to be alive, to be able to experience life and to be able to expand my knowledge. Each breath, each heartbeat, each thought, each sound I hear, everything I see, everything I feel – I am so grateful for EVERYTHING that I get to experience while being alive! Thank you Heavenly Father for the gift of life. Please help me to navigate my life and please help me to keep my body healthy so I may more fully serve thee!

~~~~~~

Rainbow

This can be offered to those that are at a level 13; however, just because they are at a level 13 that does not mean it is appropriate for them to have this connection. This is a very holy light that is offered and it requires a deep commitment to keeping our thoughts clean. A practitioner may muscle test to determine whether or not it is appropriate for a client to join in this connection.

Close your eyes and envision a world full of light. Within this light was prepared a region of darkness. **Now envision a rainbow of light surrounding the earth. This light is captured** by a multi-dimension figure and bounces off the neighboring energy rays. When this ray touches an object the object comes alive. Imagine this rainbow of light filled with the energy of the earth, the angels, God and all of creation. Focus on joining this rainbow by shining the light from each of your chakras, which will create your own rainbow. Extend your rainbow to the heavenly rainbow.

When we see a picture within our minds, this picture tends to control the manner in which we think. When these pictures are pure and righteous leading to holy thoughts, this rainbow is drawn to you. When these pictures and thoughts are negative, the rainbow is altogether too holy to remain, instead that region of darkness is invited and, thus, the region grows. This region has grown very large and strong in the recent years, so much that the world is dark with only small glimmers of light. The strength of the darkness is overpowering to even those who think they are in the light, but the darkness has become a part of them and, thus, diming their light almost to no existence. The light is powerful and creates a contagious effect. As you shine this light, the intention must be clear: your heart full of the love our Father has for all our brothers and sisters.

~~~~~~

Healing Light

Note: This is best done following a "full release" of negative energy. This is particularly important when dealing with intense illness within the body. This may not be necessary for all people.

This light will immediately break down the particles that cause you such discomfort and then allow the elements to convert the tissue into the nutrients your body needs. Do this while in the sun, lying on your back and visualizing the beam of light gently entering into your body.

Visualization: Focus on a beam of light coming from the heavens and into your body (or specific portion of your body that you desire to be healed).

Invite it in as this light obeys God's plan of free will. It will enter and immediately begin working and reorganizing the molecules within this tissue. Allow time for this to occur, be patient and allow peace to flow through your body along with deep breaths. Not just verbalizing the invitation, but welcoming this light to surge within you and into every atom.

If there's the slightest bit of resistance in your mind or subconscious, it will stop; therefore, this must be done after your release of all the energy that no longer serves you.

Be sure to release the attachments as this occurs, fully letting go.

This may take a few tries. Practice and have faith. This light represents the healing hands of Christ and healing through faith requires much work on your part. The light is loving and capable of complete healing, when you are worthy and faithful and ready – with your body no longer needing a storage facility for these energies, then you're ready.

102

Remember you are **surrounded by angels and we all work together as a team**, we are interconnected and God is our source. You may at all times be a part of this network, but during this practice of healing **you are encouraged to engage in this network and allow the angels' higher understanding to enter into you and change you from the inside out.**

You may invite your light to also join this light, stretching upwards.

Give the credit to our Father, including all your gratitude. The light also prefers to give the glory to our Father. This light comes from Father, Christ and allllllll the angels in heaven including heaven itself; therefore, it is a complete energy, complete source, and complete love.

Assignments

Energy Work:

1. Monitor any energetic wounds due to this release and heal appropriately.
2. Test for any healing compounds needed.
3. Test for any needed tapping assignment found in the Appendix.
4. Test for any remaining energies that may need to be released separately or any remaining atonement steps.
5. Continue treating any infections, toxins, parasites, and any other external sources.
6. Retest for food intolerances and only invite into your body foods that sustain life
    a. Is this good for me?
    b. Does my body want it?
    c. Can I digest it?
    d. Can I absorb it?
    e. Will this harm my body?

Homework:

1. Communicate with the body the changes that have taken place. Remind the body of its original creation. Focus on the healing hands of God upon your body now that the underlying causes have been removed. Be patient as the body heals and be aware of how your energy creates illness. Begin creating new patterns of thinking regarding the proper healing of your body with daily visualizations. Practice faith in your healing and create thought patterns regarding a body of health. Do this on your own and use your own imagery to create these patterns.
2. Practice this full release often. It is a continuous release due to the nature of life and the fact that we are always faced with adversity. Agency remains. You will still experience imperfections, but as you learn and your body learns how to process events in a Godly manner, you'll notice improved health and improved thought patterns. One day you will reflect upon the most traumatic experiences in your past and feel love and forgiveness. Be patient with yourself as this is a continuous process and takes daily effort. Practice the teachings of Christ in all your interactions and all your thoughts.

Self-Sabotage
Step Twelve

Clear Your Space

Test your client to see if these steps need to be completed before continuing. These steps are found in the Appendix. Always begin your appointments by checking for "attacks."

1. Begin by clearing the space and removing all dark influences/rebellious spirits
2. Remove Self-Destructive Tools of Dark Influences
3. Remove Mind Subconscious suggestions
4. Remove Intimidation Energy
5. Ask for shields of protection

~~~~~~

Healing Compound

There are five elements in nature that can be combined to form a powerful energetic healing compound. The energies that comprise the five elements can vary depending upon the body's needs. Muscle testing can be used to identify the components necessary for each element. Before utilizing the five elements compound, we strongly recommend practicing the basic compounds first. The guidance for using healing energetic compound is can be found with the book The Spirit Code: Compounds and Charts.

Energy Work: Invite and absorb these 5 elements into your meridian and to be distributed throughout your body for a certain amount of time. (Muscle test the most appropriate amount of days)

1. **Love** – all spiritual and all healthy energies – **synergistically combine**
2. **Earth** – Magnesium + Nickel + Yttrium + Iridium + Rhenium + Arsenic + Hafnium + #122 + #124 – **invite**
3. **Wind** – Hydrogen + Nitrogen + Oxygen + Oxygen (**merge** these four) **and then** add Helium and **merge**. This molecule will look like: H N O2 He
4. **Fire** – from the sun: Polarity magnetic connection energetic wave
   a. Take a small portion (fraction) of the energetic wave out of the whole: F 73.7 & V 28.3 – **combine**
   b. And elements from the sun: #762 + #822 + #2,246 – combine
5. **Water** – Ionized Water

Energy Work: Muscle test to see if the body needs an additional healing compound before continuing so the proper healing energy is available.

~~~~~~

Healing the Body

The body is created perfectly; however, the body can become damaged. The cells and nerve damage can become permanent, leading to chronic illness. The cause of this damage can be from an accident, emotional energies, curse/sabotage, inheritance, toxin, etc. As we age, there are many influences from poor diets and food additives, to toxins within the body, and all sorts of external influences. The body's cells become so damaged, the body no longer knows how to heal itself. This is where the spirit comes into play. The spirit does know how to heal the body. We are going to assist the spirit in teaching the body how to heal. The question is - is your body worthy of the spirit? Are you ready to see who you truly are? You are not your body. Your spirit is who you are. Your body is simply a temple to house your spirit. Once you recognize the truth and allow your spirit to shine, your body can begin to heal.

Energy work: muscle test all the locations of the body experiencing illness one by one. Ask the body these questions.

1. Is it 100% within God's will for healing to occur.
    a. No: what percentage is it within God's will to heal?
2. Is the cause of this illness/injury still present?
    a. If no: then the body is ready to heal.
    b. If yes: muscle test the cause and do the proper release based on the Spirit Code program.
        i. Note: At this point, the client has likely done a full release of negative emotions. If the cause is due to emotions, it is likely due to a live energy that will continue to be created until a lifestyle change is made. Muscle test to see what percentage of the remaining energy caused the damage to the body. For instance, if a person has eczema due to multiple energies and all but one of them have been released then they body may be capable of healing a high percentage. So just because a small portion remains, do not become discouraged by this.
3. Does the body know how to heal itself?
4. Does the spirit know how to heal the body?
5. Does the body have access to the proper healing energies?

Visualization: Close your eyes and imagine yourself walking on a cloud; within this cloud there is an entire galaxy. As the universe stretches far and expands wide, you can see all of the bits and pieces of this star scape that your body is created from. Your spirit possesses a grand knowledge, whereas one can only comprehend a minute portion of the knowledge your spirit possesses. If your spirit was given the same respect and responsibilities as your body, you would be capable of walking on water, just as Christ did. Now at this time, this is an unnecessary talent and one should not expect an unnecessary feat, unless your life depended upon it. The point is;

your body can learn from your spirit. Do not short your body the experience, knowledge or potential of the spirit. When you allow the spirit to guide, you will find yourself led down a path towards true righteousness. The mysteries of his kingdom are made available with pure intent. If it is your desire with a pure heart to learn more it will be made available to you.

While you are in this cloud, look around at the nature of your own existence as you are not standing upon flat ground. How can one exist when not experiencing gravity? And when time holds no restrictions? This goes to show how many times the brain will short circuit the spirit's capacity. Look around this cloud and allow the breath to come into your body along with the elements of the cloud. Each breath invites in the cloud into your being until the entire cloud has been invited into your spirit body. Observe others within this cloud being offered the same experience. Now that the cloud is fully within you, look down and see that you are very high above the city you live in. Take a leap of faith and jump out of the clouds and allow your spirit to fly swiftly with graceful intent. Trust in your ability to fly. As you feel the air on your face there is no fear, simply freedom. You may travel wherever you desire by simply focusing your thought on the arrival. Imagine soaring through the air free as a bird without the laws of physics weighing you down to the earth; simply allow the spirit to soar as you once did before gaining a body. The mind and body may be afraid of falling or afraid of heights or afraid of flying, but the spirit has no fear. This time the spirit deserves to be without fear and simply lead the way for the body. Focus on a destination. If you wish to visit an exotic island or swim in the sea, this is your opportunity to experience self-care for your spirit. (Pause frequently for them to experience their journey.)

Now, focus on somewhere less exotic, somewhere you can serve others. Somewhere people need help, maybe somewhere people are suffering. Find a purpose and perform an act of service for others as this is the true happiness your spirit desires. Maybe you can travel to Africa where children are starving. Maybe you can travel to a Muslim country where people are suffering. Maybe you can travel to the tip of Everest where travelers are attempting to reach the summit. You can go anywhere that people need you. There is no limit, there is no planetary limitations either if you wish to soar out of this galaxy even. But find a location where you can serve others. (Pause again for these contemplations.)

After you have completed this journey, return to the cloud. Find yourself surrounded by many others who are doing the same. Now exhale out the cloud and return it to the atmosphere above the city. Continue exhaling until all the cloud matter has been released. This is very important that this cloud matter is returned; do not keep this within you. There are two reasons why – one your spirit will not fully rejoin your body, and therefore, healing will not be attainable. Two – your spirit will not be offered this opportunity again if the gift is not returned. Now focus upon your body once again and you will be immediately be reunited.

Healing the body is a simple task based upon your faith. There are many techniques and all are worthy in their own respect; however, the spirit must merge outward with the flesh, teaching it and communicating its knowledge of the hierarchy of God's kingdom. You may focus upon your body; however, focus upon the universe, the galaxy and the Milky Way for proper guidance, as you are made up of its glorious creations. Seeking a oneness with all of God's creations, while living in peace and harmony with one another offers a safe space for the body to properly heal. As a spirit you can fly anywhere. You can do anything. However without this body you will see the many restrictions placed upon you. You cannot communicate with people who are suffering, you cannot feed the starving, you cannot free the captured and imprisoned. Your body offers opportunities to interact and serve in ways the spirit cannot. However the spirit is "WHO" you truly are. The body is simply a vessel. The spirit is what feels emotions, thinks, remembers, and possesses all the gifts of the heavens. The body cannot survive without the spirit and yet the spirit cannot succeed without the body. Open up your heart and feel this mutual respect for the body and for the spirit as each possess divine gifts. Invite your spirit to merge outward with the flesh and become one in spirit, mind and body as this mutual respect offers a higher knowledge of God's creations. When the spirit merges outward towards the flesh and becomes one, this is an act of obedience towards God as the spirit and body are created to function as one flesh. However, we tend to separate the two due to unrighteousness. The spirit is holy beyond measure and the flesh is imperfect.

Invite cobalt into your feet and up through your legs, this will ground you so this practice doesn't drain your energy. Now place your hands in front of you and imagine a bolt of electrical energy between your hands. This will take some practice. You will be able to feel this bolt of electrical energy bouncing slowly or rapidly between your hands. Have faith in your spirit's ability to control matter. Once you can feel this energy between your hands and you can visualize it, and then you are ready to use this energy. Take your time on this step as you cannot continue until this energy is being properly harnessed.

Now place your hands with your right hand at the top of your crown chakra and your left hand at your root chakra. (Top of the head and the base of your tailbone.) And leave this bolt of electrical energy within the center of your being to be used for the purpose of healing.

Strengthen your relationship with Father and Mother and rely wholly upon their love as they are the source of this knowledge and strength that feeds your spirit. When you are ready, you will be encircled in a ray of light originating from your spirit within. Now shine this light upwards towards God. In this moment ask God in prayer to shine His light originating from the heavens down upon you as it is a mutual light filled with healing energy. Offer a prayer unto your Heavenly Parents and ask for this healing light to be offered unto you and share in this mutual respect, gratitude and love for the Savior and your own creation. (Pause)

Until your body is aware of how this healing energy is meant to repair the body it will be surrounded by the nutritional benefits it needs while lacking the knowhow. Your body is now surrounded and being fully saturated in all types of healing energy, now it is time to teach the body how to utilize this energy for the proper restoration of the original creation of your body.

Your spirit is a divine being fully capable of eternal life. However, the limitations of the flesh and the blessings of the flesh tend to overcomplicate the natural law. This is a simple solution where the spirit leads the flesh and takes its place as the royal child of God with whom your true destiny lies. Your worth and your value are limitless, with potential originating from

God Himself. Step into this power and take upon yourself the crown of glory as it is offered to you for your righteousness.

Remove the binds of this earth. See yourself from beginning to end; the beginning of your creation as a spirit child of God, all the way until you are resurrected in your perfect glory. Your life does not exist only from birth of your flesh until the death of your flesh. Your existence lasts much longer. Open your mind and push past the barriers and restrictions of your mortality. You are a child of God and that existence comes with a divine purpose. Your purpose in life ultimately requires a pursuit of God's will to achieve your true calling, not in your understanding, but in His. Invite God to show you your true purpose here in life. Say a prayer and ask God to communicate to you this divine purpose. (Pause)

If this purpose is one you wish to achieve, it is recognized you will need a body of health to fully accomplish this calling. When your focus is in the right place, for the right purposes, and for the divine nature of your spirit; then your spirit will freely share this healing technique. Now ask your spirit to teach your body how to heal, reconstruct, regenerate, break down, and remove all remnants of darkness. Ask your spirit to assist the body in the knowledge of God's plan and God's creation of this perfect body. Invite your spirit to become one with your body and mind so that all may fully find peace and healing in God's tender care. Imagine all of your cells opening up and submitting fully to the spirit. Imagine these cells allowing the healing journey to regenerate to their perfect original form. Witness the energy within your body being fully recognized and welcomed into each and every atom. The atoms in your body are living, they are full of energy and they are intelligent. Ask your spirit to communicate to each atom how to function, work together, heal and regenerate as the cause of illness has been removed and repented from. Invite the body to use all the healing energy, compounds, 5 elements, and electrical energy to assist in the healing process as it is being taught by the spirit. Focus on this occurring within your body and have complete faith in your body's ability to heal with the instruction of your spirit. Focus upon each area of your body that is experiencing symptoms, illness or distress one by one. Do not guide this or limit it based upon your mortal understanding for the spirit's wisdom far exceeds your mind. (Pause for deep contemplation and for healing to occur for five minutes.)

Now take your hands and place them upon your crown and root chakra and remove this bolt of electrical energy by inviting it back into your hands. Place your hands in front of your body and offer this energy back to the earth with loving gratitude. Be sure to release this electrical energy. These steps can be repeated as often as necessary however this electrical energy is a tool meant to be used in short increments.

Focus on the healing hands of God upon your body; healing every part of your body and bringing it back to its proper function. Allow this healing to continue, throughout your day. Communicate to your body the changes that have taken place. Remind your body of its original creation and the proper functioning of every atom, every cell, every organ, and all other components that form your body wherever illness has occurred. Communicate these truths to your body: it is safe to function properly, I don't need to be sick to be loved, I can accomplish all that is required of me, I have the strength to overcome all obstacles that come my way, I desire complete health to accomplish all that God has for me, I remind my body of its original creation, and proper function as it was created perfectly by God to house my spirit during my mortal years. Now close your eyes and imagine your body in its perfect creation. See yourself full of light, health, and positive energy. Focus on this image daily and share this healing light freely.

Focus on your thoughts and the worthiness of the thoughts that come into your mind. Practice maintenance by keeping your space cleared of influences. Practice your healthy self-talk and affirmations continuously. Direct your thoughts onto a more holy understanding for your existence. Take a deep breath and feed yourself life giving thoughts. Imagine all the most positive outcomes of each trial you are currently experiencing. Imagine these one by one and focus on the best potential. Then allow God to increase the potential of each of these events as you allow more positive change to occur.

> Doctrine and Covenants 122:7 "And if thou shouldst be cast into the pit, or into the hands of murderers, and the sentence of death passed upon thee; if thou be cast into the deep; if the billowing surge conspire against thee; if fierce winds become thine enemy; if the heavens gather blackness, and all the elements combine to hedge up the way; and above all, if the very jaws of hell shall gape open the mouth wide after thee, know thou, my son, that all these things shall give thee experience, and shall be for thy good."

~~~~~~

Clean-Up

Deep in the drama of contention or life's trials, it is hard to remember how to climb out. It's as if blinders filter out all reason and we are only left with despair. It is expected that you'll experience some struggles as we are all imperfect mortals. In general, once you experience an "attack," you will recognize it right away, because after removing all this darkness you'll feel the difference immediately. You may feel as though you have lost all progress and there is little hope for you. So here are a few "clean-up" steps you can take on your own once you become familiar with the process. Teach your client how to do these basic maintenance steps. Always "bring to light" all energies/spirits/cords prior to any steps. Also be aware that others bring their own influences into your home and there are many possible causes to "attacks", do not fret when this occurs. Simply clean-up and move on.

1. Become aware of the rebellious spirits influencing you and taking away your ability to control your own emotions. Do not be afraid to muscle test and cast out the rebellious spirits.
    a. Put your right arm to the square – "In the name of Jesus Christ I command all rebellious spirits to depart immediately and I seal any and all portals. I detach these cords, I cut these cords with the sword of the rebellion, I release and remove these cords.

2. Prayer. This is a big one. Pray, pray, pray. This is hard to do when contention is boiling, but stop and pray for help to turn the situation around. You are not alone and you do not have to fight off the negative influences alone.

3. Consider the other person's intentions. We all have reasons for doing certain things. We all make mistakes. We do not have to force others to see things the way we see them. Be patient and forgiving. "Soften your heart to your partner's intentions as you are both in this trial of life together. Always choose the view least obscured by imperfections or ill worded opinions." – Healing from Above Book One by Alexandria and Calvin

4. Be aware of the negative cords attached to you and their influence. Then remove them safely.
   a. Command rebellious spirits off the cords in a manner similar to step 1a.
   b. "I untie all knots that can be untied. I send love, peace and the healing light of the atonement into these cords and convert all cords that can be converted."
   c. All remaining cords – "I detach all remaining cords, I cut these cords with the flaming sword, I release these cords and I remove these cords. (Use the sword chart in The Spirit Code program to be specific with the cutting tool.)

5. Check for a broken heart and open energetic wounds and seal them. You may need assistance with this one until it becomes familiar. The entire process is in the spirit code program – the energy that caused the wound may need to be released and if that energy is living further steps may need to be addressed. Here's a very simplified basic step:
   a. "I ask for the healing stick to seal any open wounds. I invite my heart/spirit back into one piece. I invite my spirit back into my body. I zip up my spirit, mind and body." (visualize it being healed and it will be more effective)

6. Check to see if you put up a wall for protection and actively choose to remove it or convert it into something more loving.
   a. This may need to be done similar to step 1 wall removal. However, once removing the rebellious spirit/contract; then you can convert it into something more positive such as a tree of life within your home.
   b. When working with a contracted spirit always offer them 3 choices – repent, depart or be cast out. Always remove their chains/cords and wash the contract in living waters or burn it with lava.

7. Check for mind subconscious suggestions and tools of dark influence and remove them.
   a. Refer to the Appendix for these steps, pages 118 and 119.

8. Do a tapping sequence to balance the hormones. Tapping is taught in Step Six and the sequences are written in the Appendix.

9. Check for any dark energies and release them as taught in The Spirit Code program.

10. Be aware of your self-talk and practice self-care. Stand in the mirror and say affirmations until you feel a shift and no longer resist these words, "I love myself exactly as I am right now. I love myself the same as God loves me. I am confident and strong. I am a royal child of God with infinite worth."

11. Invite healing energies into your space. For example, "I invite and absorb into my meridian a continuous flow of peace, Godly love, the light of Christ, patience, tolerance, self-love and forgiveness. I ask these energies to be distributed throughout my body and energy fields for the next_____ hours/days."

12. Ask for your shields to be returned in the manner previously created. Strengthen them with the love of God. Shields are attached to your spirit which means they remain

permanent until you experience an "attack" and then they will drop as they have become weakened.

As you can see, much more can be added to the steps listed. Feel free to add your own steps. You can print them off so you have a quick reference to them until you have them thoroughly memorized. Keep them simple, so it will not feel as if you need to climb a mountain when there is really just a small hill with angels escorting you.

~~~~~~

Maintenance

When your mind is polluted it is best to unload it a bit at a time and replace the pollution with Godly images/words/thoughts. Due to the nature of life, it stands to reason you may need to repeat some of these steps often in your life. You are experiencing opportunities for growth every day and growth requires resistance. There are some preventative measures that can assist in keeping your home's vibrations high, keeping your mind clean, and keeping attacks cleared.

1. When you have visitors into your home, be aware of the potential of influences tagging along. When there is contention, be aware there will be influences on the newly formed negative cords.
2. Choose your music wisely as it will repeat in your mind and sometimes make it difficult to hear the still small voice of the Holy Ghost. Some music can have the opposite effect and invite in the enemy.
3. Limit your exposure to television and choose your entertainment wisely. Do you choose enlightenment or entertainment? When inappropriate images play in your mind, work on removing the pollution through energy work, repentance, and prayer. Then invite the Holy Ghost back into the home.
4. Refrain from violent expressions of emotions and focus on your true emotions and how to express yourself in a healthy manner. If you find it difficult to express yourself, pause and step into the shoes of the other person to see things from their perspective or better yet – step into God's perspective.
5. Incorporate all the steps and guidance offered in these 12 steps daily. When you find yourself slipping into the victim cycle, quickly recognize what needs to change and take action. Keep your environment cleared and follow the Spirit's promptings.
6. Shift your perspective of your creation and existence. Begin seeing the earth, food, nutrition, water, animals, trees, life in all forms – as creations of a loving God. Become one with all of God's creations by forming a deep respect for all of creation.
7. Play uplifting music in the kitchen to raise the vibrations of the food and water. Invite food and water into your body to sustain life. Imagine the life cycle of the food/water before it enters your body. Ask God to bless your food to offer life for this body God has given you for the purpose of properly nourishing your body.
8. Begin seeing your spirit's worth within this amazing body God has formed just for you. Allow your spirit to lead your life and form a deep respect for this body you have the opportunity to care for. Shift your perspective for the body you have been offered and begin seeing the changes naturally take form.

9. Direct your thoughts towards positive uplifting words, emotions and desires. Begin with self-talk and work outward towards other people. Be aware your energy affects others.

10. Pray for others, especially your enemies. This healing gift will heal from the inside out. "If you walk with the Savior long enough, you will learn to see everyone as a Child of God with limitless potential regardless of what his/her past may have been and if you continue walking with the Savior you will develop another gift He has; the ability to help people see that potential in themselves and so to repent." –Henry B. Eyring

11. Offer service to others. Focus your attention outwards. We are all in this trial of life together, let us take this journey together. Begin seeing others from the inside; for whom they are in their heart and love as our Savior loves.

12. Offer gratitude for everything; from your breath to the creation of the planet. Focus on the lifecycle of the other individuals you meet to the food you eat. We are all one.

13. Practice visualizing outcomes of your life in tune with God's ultimate plan for you. Remove the need for temporal perfection and focus on a more eternal progression. See yourself living your life for God and His mission for all of His children.

14. Love yourself. Speak life affirming words at all times towards yourself and others. The Savior gave a commandment to love one another. However to truly offer love to another, you must first love yourself. This life you are living is an amazing gift from God, you are created in His image, and you are a product of His hands. Love is of God. Take care of this life you are living, because it is your only chance you have to be alive! If there is discord in any area of your life; seek improvement and create a new outcome.

15. Watch your energy and words towards others. Remove judgment, criticism, and gossip. Offer others agency to be themselves. Love others in their imperfections and swiftly forgive. There is no need to change the opinions of others, simply love them as they are.

16. Remember Christ is our Brother. We have the same potential as He. Never remain complacent in your growth. Do not listen to the enemy as he seeks to make you forget WHO YOU ARE and where your potential lies.

17. Live your life in the manner Christ lived His life. He has come to this earth to show us how to love. Create a life that is centered in God and you will see how everything around you begins to change shape. Your relationships, your career, your family dynamics, your patience, and your mental/physical health. Allow Him to teach you how to love.

18. Repent daily until your thoughts are worthy of God's presence in all aspects. Remain humble, teachable, and kind. Repentance is not limited to sinning against the 10 commandments, but against God's higher law. Do not excuse these sins and confuse this with being imperfect. God's gift of grace comes to those humble enough to receive.

19. Just because you cannot see the angels doesn't mean they aren't there. The same goes for the healing hands of Christ. There is opposition in all things. Be aware who you are inviting into your presence through your thoughts, words, and actions.

20. Energy is real... You are energy and your body is living. Your body is designed to heal itself naturally. Create an environment for your body to heal by removing the darkness that's polluting your body and then maintain the light of Christ. Healing takes time; be patient.

The Light of Christ

The amount of individuals upon the planet living a Christ-like centered life is surprisingly low. We may believe in Christ, but do we truly live completely in the manner He taught us by His example? If this light goes out completely, the world would fall into chaos. Test what percentage you are shining the light of Christ from within you. Your light is a result of your thoughts, actions, and energy.

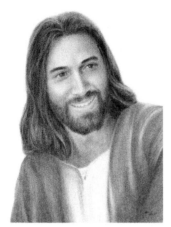

Focus upon Jesus Christ and ask for the light within you to open up towards God and shine to its maximum potential. Invite your light from within to open up and pour forth the full magnitude of its creation. Imagine all the angels of heaven are interconnected and "one" with God. This light surrounds the earth and is available to all those who are ready to release the need for negativity, invite this light to merge with your light. Continue focusing on the love of God and imagine your light growing brighter and brighter. As you shift your life to a more Christ-like perspective you will see this light growing brighter and stronger too.

Always seek to increase your light through your daily thoughts, service and energy. Be open to the light coming forth from the heavens to merge with the light from your spirit.

Positive Cords with Everybody

At Level 27 or higher we can create positive cords with all people on earth.

1. First, we already need to be connected to Heavenly Father, Jesus Christ and the Holy Ghost.
2. Offer positive cords filled with God's LOVE to be created between you and ALL people on earth. (Optional: include those to be born in the future and all the angels in heaven.)
3. Convert any negative cords into positive cords by inviting in the love of God, atonement energy, forgiveness and understanding. Then shine such a powerful loving light through the cords which forces all unclean spirits to depart. Visualize this until it is complete.
4. Ask for the lens of kindness into the cords… I form a permanent lens of kindness for the ways in which I view myself and others. I ask that the lens magnify my good qualities and the qualities I see in others. I ask this lens to provide clarity and understanding to undesirable qualities.

Spiritual Senses

There are 38 Spiritual Senses available to us as full grown mortal beings at this time. An infant is born with 72 functioning spiritual senses. Most mothers feel a strong sense of protection due to the hyper awareness of this sacred innocence. As their senses die off, a mother may actually feel this and mourn without knowing why. An adult has the capacity to have 38 functioning spiritual senses while in this mortal body. Each of the senses available to your spirit concludes in behalf of one frequency resonating tone 7.83 hertz. This balance begins with a simple tone of patience, love and respect. When you "tap" (also known as EFT), you do essentially the opposite emotion of what created the imbalance, while stimulating the meridian points?... So awakening these senses to their full functioning capability, will be accomplished much the same. Awakening a spiritual sense is **faith-based and action motivated**. Speaking up for God takes humility, dedication and spiritual strength. Individuals over a level 52 are spiritually ready to take this step. Awareness of this ability is just as important as the senses themselves. The more you seek, the more ye shall find. This is critical for your progression – the agency of mankind revolves around pursuing truths. Complacency leads to its own form of dogma.

This is a simple decision and desire. Simply wanting these senses for your own personal gain will not be permitted. The Lord knows your heart; those with a true righteous desire will be granted this gift which has been neglected.

1. Note: Level 52 and above
2. Note: Spiritual senses resonate at 7.83 hertz – is more of a result of living in a healthy manner, spiritually, mentally, emotionally and physically
3. **First,** becoming aware of the existence of the extra-sensory perception and 38 total spiritual senses
4. **Second,** begin with a tone of patience, love and respect
5. **Third,** being committed to speaking up for God
6. **Fourth,** being humble, dedicated and spiritually strong enough to receive and follow through

Remember: Awakening a spiritual sense is faith-based and action motivated.

Note: If your spiritual senses exceed 38 or your level exceeds 100, you are most likely a healer, guardian, awoken angel, protector or defender. These are simply special callings we are ordained to perform in these latter days before the return of Jesus Christ. There are others, but this is all we have learned at this time.

Grand Finale

You are never done. There is no grand finale saying, "you are perfect and will never experience a difficult day," or "you will never experience trials," or "you will never experience illness." This life is an opportunity to grow, but with growth comes trials. Now you have a better perspective and you have taken the steps necessary to change your life. These practices must remain a daily part of life. Continue to shift your thoughts to the Savior and keeping your influences pure. Over time you will see these changes have become who you are. You will notice how much you have grown. Your body will begin healing and improving and as circumstances present themselves, you'll see how much your thoughts influence you.

Always work towards your higher goal in this life. Set your monthly goals and daily goals each to align with your higher purpose. **Set yourself up for success** in the manner this manual has laid out. Always turn to God for further guidance and assistance. Your progression requires growth from your comfort zones which involves constantly seeking to improve yourself. Never remain complacent, always seek a higher understanding and hold yourself accountable for your actions. Keep the atonement close to your heart as this life is a constant opportunity for growth. You are never alone as Christ is always walking by your side.

There is a master's program for those who wish to continue on this journey. Prior to continuing on; master these 12 steps until they become a part of you and it is your passion. There is no reward for completion, work these steps often. Your results will be contingent upon your readiness, obedience, patience, faith, and MOST importantly God's will.

One day very soon, the events prophesied in the book of Revelations will begin prior to the return of our Savior. These events have been prophesied as nothing short of complete destruction. We believe these events will occur in OUR lifetime. There will be suffering, sorrow, starvation, plagues, diseases, disasters, and difficulties beyond our current comprehension. The question you must ask yourself is; are you ready? When these events occur and you lose loved ones and witness horrific sights; can you heal? When your current trials are miniscule to the trials that have yet to come; can you still have joy in your heart? Can you forgive in the face of the trials? Can you bring others up while you are hurting inside? Can you sacrifice your comforts for the return of the Savior? Can you sing and shout with the armies of heaven? Are you worthy right now to be in the presence of the prophets and apostles of old? Are you stable enough in your healing journey to place all your faith in God for your survival? Can you sing and find joy in the midst of suffering? Is your faith strong enough to rely upon God and not the arms of flesh?

There is much to learn from how Christ radiated love even while he was being tortured and crucified. He didn't wait until years after to process His healing. He experienced the journey and in the midst of suffering; He chose love over hate, forgiveness over resentment, and healing over suffering. We must live our lives now, in the manner Christ lived so that when we are faced with trials beyond measure, we can respond in the same manner.

We've learned in the scriptures that God gave manna to the people of Moses. He fed a thousand with one loaf of bread and a few fish. He walked on water. He healed the sick. He raised the dead. Miracles are real! They have NOT ceased, they are as accessible as the air you breathe if you only believe.

Have faith my friend. We shall make it there; when Christ shall descend with open arms. We shall travel together in this journey towards Zion. I pray you prepare yourself to handle all that shall come as none shall be without.

With our love we leave these things with you in the name of Jesus Christ, amen.

Afterword

Visit Spiritcode.net for further opportunities to learn more about energy healing, full energy releases, more tapping sequences, and much more. Or contact us at thespiritcode@gmail.com

Appendix

Clearing Your Space

Preparation: Though much can be said about clearing your space there are some basics that are essential. If you are clearing for yourself, you must be in a place where the spirit can be present not only in your heart, mind but also in your physical presence. Ideally, this would be a place where it is quiet and peaceful. Though this seems very basic, turn off mobile devices, music, TV, anything that can distract. Dedicate this time to your absolute focus.

If you are clearing for others, a wonderful thing to do is to have your space dedicated to healing. Priesthood power is inseparably connected with the power of heaven and will lay a perfect foundation for this work.

To understand clearing, we will first define what it is that can be cleared and then describe how to clear the space so further energy work can be done. A question was asked, as to why is clearing the space is needed. Consider this analogy. You are ready to make an incredible gourmet meal but the kitchen is messy. You know to have the wanted outcome for your dinner, you must be able to work in a space that is clear and free of all toxins. The same is true of energy work. You must be able to work in a space that can give the best platform for healing.

Rebellious Spirits: The term we use to group together all types of spirits who have chosen to follow Lucifer is "rebellious spirits;" this is a more complete term which includes disembodied spirits, entities, predators, deceivers, mutated etc.

Mutated spirits: These spirits are very powerful. They do not respond to the name Jesus Christ. These spirits are too powerful to remove on our own; request the assistance of some hounds to remove them. And invite the hounds to mark their territory on your shields.

Other spirits: There are many other types of spirits that do not follow after God; however, we feel that these are the most critical to address, as they are the most common. If further assistance with spirits is needed, feel free to contact us.

Cording: Positive and negative cords are very common. When removing rebellious spirits and other forms of negative energy it is important to also remove the negative cords that are connected to that spirit/energy. To remove the cords, it is important to go through the four step process; otherwise, the cords have the potential of cause energetic wounds: 1) Detach, 2) Cut, 3) Release, 4) Remove. For the cutting process several swords can be used depending upon the spirit involved. Options include the Flaming Sword, the Ice Sword, the Hellfire Sword, the Revolving sword, the **Sword of the Rebellion,** and the **Sword of Certain Limited Freedom**. The last two swords listed (in bold) each have the ability to cut all types of negative cords to rebellious spirits. There are many more that are not listed. The more specific the sword, the more effective and safe the removal will be.

Portals: Rebellious spirits utilize portals to jump from place to place. The portals must be sealed and their cords removed as well. There are several different types of portals, which will be discussed within their own document in the Spirit Code Program.

Clearing rebellious spirits and portals: It is recommended to remove the rebellious spirits and portals from a person, their home and property (land), vehicles and all items within the home.

Example #1:

1. "I bring to light all rebellious spirits and portals within and corded to me, each of my family members, my home and all items within my home."
2. (Put your right arm to the square) "In the name of Jesus Christ, I command that all rebellious spirits depart and I command that the portals created by rebellious spirits to be sealed and never again be reopened.
3. "I detach the **cords** to the rebellious spirit. I cut the cords with the Sword of the Rebellion. I release and remove the cords."

Example #2:

1. "I bring to light all rebellious spirits and portals within and corded to me, each of my family members, my home and all items within my home."
2. Give the rebellious spirit **three options**:
   a. "Repent and become an angel in training, turn your heart towards God and accept the atonement."
   b. "Or depart and leave with your own agency."
   c. Or if they choose to attack, then cast them out:
3. Casting out: (Put your right arm to the square) "All rebellious spirits that remain - In the name of Jesus Christ, I command that you depart and I command that the portals be sealed and never again be reopened."

Powerful Spirits: As mentioned above under mutated spirits some spirits do not respond to the name of Jesus Christ. There a few additional steps you can take.

- Command in the name of "Elohim, Jehovah and The Holy Ghost."
- Ask for the Sun to shine upon the rebellious spirits. And then ask for a magnifying glass to intensify the Sun's rays.
- Ask for some heavenly assistance. Warrior angels are great. There are some spirit animals that are also exceptional at removing rebellious spirits:
  - Ask for some big cats to remove them.
  - Ask for a hound to remove them. (The hounds are like the special forces when it comes to removing rebellious spirits. So don't request their assistance unless you feel as though you need to.)
    - Follow this up by asking them to "mark their territory" on your shields

There are spirits that even the hounds cannot remove. Some of those are addressed under the advanced section. Again, if further assistance with removing spirits is needed feel free to contact us.

Shields: Once everything has been cleared, instruct all of your shields to be restored.

Filling with Light: Whenever you remove a negative form of energy from a space take the time and fill it with a positive form of energy so that you can once again get the optimum advantage in your healing platform. Ask that the Light of Christ, the love of God and Truth fill the space that was once filled with darkness. Also invite the space to remember its original creation and purpose for which God made it. Note: In the energy releases the compounds and the last atonement step assist in filling this space.

Self-Destructive Tools of Dark Influence

Explanation: This term encompasses 28 types of energy that are intended to cause destruction to an individual. These tools including curses, sabotages, eggs...etc (eggs are kind of like a time released curse/sabotage). These tools are often used by rebellious spirits; however, a mortal can also use these tools without consciously realizing it. Tools are commonly cast upon individuals we have conflict with. Remember, our thoughts and intentions are powerful and they can literally cause a great amount of destruction to others.

Before removing the tools, first clear the space of the individual. This is important, because as long as the spirits are present they will continue to cast tools upon the individual. (See: Clear Your Space).

Option 1: For a more thorough process follow the steps below. This is **recommended for the initial clearing**, as there are additional benefits contained within the steps.

1. "I bring to light all of the Self-Destructive Tools of Dark Influences that are within and corded to me. I bring to light all of the rebellious spirits and portals corded to the tools and upon the cords."
2. In the name of Jesus Christ, I command all of the rebellious spirits to depart and I command that portals be sealed and never again be reopened.
3. I detach all cords to the Self-Destructive Tools.
4. I cut all cords to the Self-Destructive Tools with the Sun Sword.
5. I release and remove all cords.
6. I ask for the golden net to gather up all the Self-Destructive Tools.
7. I neutralize and defuse the frequencies and vibrations of all Self-Destructive Tools.
8. I detach, release and remove the Self-Destructive Tools.
9. I ask for a flying sword to take the golden net filled with all Self-Destructive Tools to a black hole.
10. I ask the flying sword and the golden net to then return to their place of origin.
11. I place a healing stick upon each of the imprints left from the Self-Destructive Tools."
12. Muscle test to see if there has been any poison left from the Tools. If poison remains:
    a. "I convert all poison within the spirit into white powder gold."
13. "I invite the energy of love, peace, calm, etc. into my presence." - whatever energy you desire

Option 2:

1. "I bring to light all of the Self-Destructive Tools of Dark Influences that are within and corded to me. I bring to light all of the rebellious spirits and portals corded to the tools and upon the cords."
2. In the name of Jesus Christ, I command all of the rebellious spirits to depart and I command that portals be sealed and never again be reopened.
3. I converted all of the tools and their cords into - **High Density Magnetic Plasma"**

Mind Subconscious Suggestions

Explanation: Mind subconscious suggestions comprise of 67 types of suggestions (thoughts or images) that are placed within a person's mind either by themselves, other people or rebellious spirits. By following the steps below we can effectively remove 66 types, the one that is excluded is self-created. Shifting the core beliefs will be required for a lasting removal of the self-created suggestions.

The 66 types include suggestions, such as:

- Post-hypnotic suggestions
- Subliminal messages
- Despair anchors
- Broadcast messages
- Images

Keep in mind our thoughts are very powerful. Our thoughts are a form of energy that can be projected towards other people. Casting judgment on others and labeling them have real effects that are recognized by the subconscious. Imagine how much hard it might be for a recovering alcoholic if everybody around that person labeled them as an alcoholic. We can assist others by sending positive messages instead. Reality has to play a part in this too; we can't save everyone, but we can still love everyone. Send the message of love to all that are in your presence.

Removing Mind Subconscious Suggestions:

Options #1:

For a more thorough process follow the steps below. This is **recommended for the initial clearing**, as there are multiple benefits contained within the steps.

1. Mind Subconscious Suggestions
    a. I bring to light the truth of all mind subconscious suggestions, the blocks around the transmitters and receivers, along with all of the cords, and the rebellious spirits and portals upon the cords.
        i. Remove the rebellious spirits and close the portals upon the cords
    b. I shine the Light of Truth and Happiness upon all mind subconscious suggestions. I form a permanent lens of kindness for the ways in which I view myself and others. I ask that the lens magnify my good qualities and the qualities I see in others. I ask this lens to provide clarity and understanding to undesirable qualities.
    c. I neutralize and defuse all mind subconscious suggestions
    d. I merge all subcategories of mind subconscious suggestions within each category
    e. I emulsify all categories of mind subconscious suggestions
    f. I detach the cords to the mind subconscious suggestions
    g. I cut the cords with the Sword of Understanding
    h. I choose to accept the truth by viewing all mind subconscious suggestions in their true nature

  i. I release and remove the cords

  j. I detach, release and remove all the mind subconscious suggestions

  k. I reverse the confused belief system the body has been led to participate in by shining the light of truth upon your body, mind, spirit and accepting God's perfect love for you. (There is a tangible block that is blocking the senses from feeling properly- created for protection)

    i. Detach the blocks around the transmitters and receivers

    ii. Detach the cords to the blocks / Cut the cords with a laser / Release the cords / Remove the cords

    iii. I now invite my (and/or the person's) light to outshine the darkness around the transmitters and receivers

    iv. Release the blocks / Remove the blocks

    v. We/I invite a steady flow of God's love to remind all dead transmitters and receivers of their original creation and purpose for which God created them

    vi. Gently remind the transmitters and receivers that the block is gone and that energy can flow freely

  l. "I (the healer) wish to offer my energy, strength, understanding, and complete love with you (the client). I invite you to step out of the shadows and relish in the feelings of this great love with me and all others that desire to love you." – note: it is important for the participation of both the healer and client

  m. "We/I ask for the assistance of a spiritual compass as we/I form a truth shield around my/client's mind and body. We/I ask the truth shield to filter out the lies coming from outside sources and to only invite in truth. We/I ask for this truth shield to convert the mind subconscious suggestions into these words – I am a child of God. I am valuable. I am worth it. God loves me. I am never alone. There is nobody in the whole world just like me. I am special. I am loved. I am beautiful."

Option #2:

  To simply remove these, convert them into positive thoughts of your choosing. The conversion process is unable to convert all types. Remember to bring them all to light and remove the rebellious spirits and portals that will be attached to many of them or upon the cords.

Intimidation Energy

God has created many forms of positive energy that can fill our home and surrounding space wherever we are. Unfortunately, this same energy can be turned into negative energy. As an example, when a person traps a positive energy, the energy losses its freedom. The energy becomes tainted and is turned into a negative energy. This is why we are able to convert negative energy into positive once we set it free. In the case of self-destructive tools of dark influence, we can convert the tools and their cords into high density magnetic plasma (a positive energy) once the connection to the rebellious spirits have been removed.

In the case of intimidation energy, this energy was originally created by rebellious spirits and cannot be converted into positive energy. This energy is much more intense than the negative energy that was originally created as positive energy. The weight of intimidation energy will suffocate and congest the breath of oxygen available to you. This energy is present in many homes where rebellious spirits reside.

To remove the **intimidation energy:**

1. Bring to light all intimidation energy
2. Ask for our Father in heaven to shine His light down upon you and your home to convert the air into loving rays of energy.
3. Neutralize/ Defuse the intimidation energy
4. Detach the cords / Cut with the Sword of Strength
5. Release / Remove the cords
6. Detach / Release / Remove the intimidation energy
7. Reject the intimidation energy
8. Invite motivational energy into the space, such as the spiritual energies of:
   - The pure love of God
   - Holiness to the Lord, the house of the Lord
   - Faith in His plan
   - Fully accepting the gift of God's free will
   - Faith in God to support you
   - Faith to move a mountain
   - I am a child of God
   - The divinity of my holy spirit
   - Love for all mankind
   - Forgiveness for my enemies
9. Cast the intimidation energy into the fiery pits of hell

Shields

Shields are a holy opportunity to protect your space from further influences or attacks. Shields are permanent if you intend them to be. As long as you are worthy of the shields and as long as your spirit is in one piece, they should also remain as they are an extension of your spirit. We cannot create spiritual matter; however we can work together with our spirit to create this shield. After any contention it is important to recognize the shields may have gone down and "clean-up" may be necessary. Simply clear the space and ask for the shields to be returned and then repeat initial testing.

Asking for the shield by name and closing your eyes and envisioning them being formed around the individual is successful. Always teach your client how to keep their shields in place. Being aware they are a choice and that worthiness and respect to your spirit and yourself will keep them strong.

You can also ask The Love of God to interweave in any shield to strengthen it. It will look like a golden thread that binds tighter than any shield we can create alone.

Shield Types:

1. **Basic Shield:** This is given to everyone immediately upon clearing their space.
2. **Love Shield:** This is offered between two individuals: a married couple or a parent and their children.
3. **Truth Shield**: This is to convert all negativity coming from outside sources into positive words and thoughts. "I ask for the assistance of a spiritual compass as I form a truth shield around my/client's mind and body. I ask the truth shield to filter out the lies coming from outside sources and to only invite in truth. I ask for this truth shield to convert the mind subconscious suggestions into these words – I am a child of God. I am valuable. I am worth it. God loves me. I am never alone. There is nobody in the whole world just like me. I am special. I am loved. I am beautiful."
4. **Property Shield:** This is to keep your entire home and property free of rebellious spirits.
5. **Body Armor:** This is specifically to protect you from energetic wounds created by rebellious spirits
6. **Dream Shield:** This must be done nightly to protect from nightmares until the dream dark energy is removed.
7. **Sight and Sound Shield:** This is a shield to make you invisible to rebellious spirits and its sound proof.

Affirmations

Affirmations are simple as you choose to be consciously in control of your thoughts. They are short, powerful statements. When you say them or think them or even hear them, they become the thoughts that create your reality. Affirmations, then, are your conscious thoughts. To affirm means to say something positively. It means to declare firmly and assert something to be true. Test which ones your client needs and how often in order to produce a new positive core belief.

1. I am love.
2. I forgive myself for all the mistakes I have made.
3. I am the architect of my life; I build its foundation and choose its contents.
4. Happiness is a choice. I base my happiness on my own accomplishments and the blessings I've been given.
5. Today, I am brimming with energy and overflowing with joy.
6. As I listen, may my heart be touched and my faith increased.
7. I forgive those who have harmed me in my past and peacefully detach from them.
8. I am conquering my illness; I am defeating it steadily each day.
9. A river of compassion washes away my anger and replaces it with love.
10. I possess the qualities needed to be extremely successful.
11. I am courageous and I stand up for myself.
12. My thoughts are filled with positivity and my life is plentiful with prosperity.
13. I wake up today with strength in my heart and clarity in my mind.
14. My future is an ideal projection of what I envision now.
15. My ability to conquer my challenges is limitless; my potential to succeed is infinite.
16. I am breaking the cycle. The past has no power over me anymore.
17. I replace my anger with understanding and compassion.
18. Many people look up to me and recognize my worth; I am admired.
19. Creative energy surges through me and leads me to new and brilliant ideas.
20. I offer an apology to those affected by my anger.
21. I choose to find hopeful and optimistic ways to look at life.
22. I acknowledge my own self-worth; my confidence is soaring.
23. I have the power to change myself.
24. Miracles really do accompany me in my life.
25. I turn my faith into action.
26. I build my life upon a safe and sure foundation.
27. I radiate positive energy.
28. I radiate beauty, charm, and grace.
29. I am strong. I can do this. I believe in myself.
30. I love my body; this incredible and complex vessel is me. I am in awe of my body's ability to heal, to nurture, to transform, to love and to flourish with vibrant health and divine energy. I see the perfection in every one of my cells and honor this physical vehicle that I have been blessed with.
31. I am in complete harmony with my body.
32. I believe in the power of positive thinking.

Affirmations

33. When I experience an intense emotion, I acknowledge my feelings and allow the energy to flow back out of my body.
34. I live in the present and am confident of the future.
35. I soften my heart to the intentions of others as we are all in this trial of life together. I choose the view least obscured by imperfections or ill worded opinions.
36. I consciously choose to let go of old patterns and I invite my mind to form new thoughts and patterns which will lead towards true happiness in life.
37. I love change and easily adjust myself to new situations.
38. I am at peace with my past as it formed me into who I am today.
39. I am energetic and enthusiastic. Confidence is my nature.
40. I accept and offer the gift of free will to all others in this life. With this gift of agency, I also offer respect and peace for our differences as individuals.
41. I choose to see the good in others.
42. I love and accept every inch of my body exactly as it is right now.
43. I am grateful for the gift of free will that is given to everybody.
44. I shift my opinions of others and choose to only speak and think loving thoughts towards others.
45. I take responsibility for my own feelings and reactions.
46. I am confident in myself and I do not need the approval of others because I know the truth about myself and who I am. I love myself.
47. I trust my body and I no longer choose to hold onto negative energy as it does not serve me.
48. I fully accept myself and know that I am worthy of great things in life.
49. I am more than capable of bringing my dreams to life.
50. I give myself permission to be and do what I want.
51. I am whole, complete and perfect just as I am.
52. Positive energy flows through me; each cell of my being is awake and alive with joy.
53. I release limiting beliefs and know that miracles happen daily.
54. I deserve nutrition. The nourishment I choose to put into body offers me strength, stamina, mental clarity and joy. I deserve to eat.
55. Food is safe and eating is safe. I enjoy eating surrounded by my family and friends.
56. My body is a reflection of the choices I make. I choose to be healthy; I choose to exercise my body, strengthen my body, nourish my body and speak loving words to my body. I love my body.
57. I am amazing, unique and worthwhile just as I am today. I am ever growing, ever changing, ever moving forward. I am an amazing individual worthy of respect, love and joy. I am walking my own path at my own pace. I know the truth about myself and the opinions of others do not change my belief that I am perfect just as I am in this very moment.
58. It is safe to recover from my addictions.
59. My self-worth is growing every single day and every single moment.
60. Letting go of the past is easy as I welcome new, fresh and vital experiences into my life.
61. My thoughts are the creation of my belief system therefore I choose to believe the very best in myself.

Affirmations

62. The life I lead has been created completely by my daily choices. Every thought, memory, belief and choice has led me towards my current experiences. I know this life is a compilation of my experiences. Therefore I choose to love my life and forgive those who have caused me distress.

63. My past represents opportunities to grow. I no longer see my past as stumbling blocks, instead I choose to see opportunities to grow and move forward. I choose to move forward and learn from the past to improve my future.

Spiritual Affirmations

64. I love myself the same as God loves me.

65. I love my body exactly as it is right now.

66. I am a royal Child of God of Infinite Worth.

67. Making, keeping, and rejoicing in my covenants is evidence that the Atonement of Jesus Christ is truly written in my heart.

68. I am blessed as I feel gratitude for the Atonement of Jesus Christ.

69. I dedicate myself to a life-long quest to become more like the Savior.

70. I feel of God's love and compassion.

71. Jesus Christ is the source of my hope.

72. I choose to fill myself up with the pure love of Christ for all mankind including myself.

73. I choose to form righteous thoughts for my brothers and sisters while focusing on Christ-like love.

74. I am so grateful for this body that my loving Father in Heaven created to house my spirit during this trial of my life.

75. I know my body was created perfectly and is designed by God to heal and protect me. Therefore I desire to function as a team with my body, my mind and my spirit.

76. I know I am valuable, I know I am a child of God and I know my existence matters.

77. I will only allow others to treat me with kindness. When I am faced with any contention, I choose to respond lovingly, as my Savior has taught me.

78. I choose to speak kindly of others at all times, the way my loving Savior has taught me to treat my brothers and sisters. I also choose to speak and think only loving words and thoughts about myself as I am a royal child of God and I deserve the utmost respect.

79. I offer unconditional love to my Creator and I offer unconditional love to all my brothers and sisters. I am honored to be a Royal Child of God of Infinite Worth.

80. I commit to live my life in accordance with the commandments of God.

81. Father in Heaven loves me and He created me perfectly to experience joy according to His plan. Father has a plan for me and the creation is for my happiness.

82. As I face trials in my life, I choose a path free of an entanglement of contentious thorns. I will instead shine my light so bright that all may see and feel of the eternal love radiating from within, which comes from my Father in Heaven.

83. I choose to stay connected to my loving Father in Heaven throughout my life. I invite my Father in Heaven and my Savior Jesus Christ into my heart and I allow them to see me fully and completely.

Affirmations

84. As a Child of God, love is my birthright. I have an endless supply of love.

85. My Father in Heaven created my body in His image. What a gift and a blessing I have been entrusted. I choose to care for this body and spirit through healthy thinking; healthy habits, clean eating, exercising and I will always offer pure love to this gift. I love my body!

86. My thoughts are loving and positive as I desire to be more like my Savior Jesus Christ.

87. I have been called to live in the last days to prepare the world for the return of Jesus Christ and because of this sacred calling; I will prepare myself and dedicate my life to my Savior. I know He lives and loves me, I also choose to love myself and others the way God loves me.

88. The Savior is returning to the earth and I dedicate my time and life to Him. I choose sacred thoughts that lead me towards righteousness so I may be found worthy in His presence. I want to live the higher law where even my thoughts are worthy of His presence. I guard my thoughts with the armor of God.

89. I humble myself to God's will and He loves me unconditionally. I trust God with my past, present and future.

90. I am worthy of God's love, I accept His love, I share His love, I resonate His love and I know I deserve His love. Others in my presence can feel His love as His light shines from my soul.

91. I am ever growing, ever progressing, ever changing, ever improving and ever striving to become more like my Savior Jesus Christ.

92. I align my path in life with God's will as I choose to walk the straight and narrow way. When I experience any distress, I choose to humble myself to God and continue on the path towards righteousness.

93. Every thought that comes from God floods into my life freely. I choose to barricade all negativity that comes from the adversary.

94. I choose thoughts that resonate God's perfect love. I know my body and soul are perfect creations of God and therefore they deserve only Godly thoughts to experience complete harmony with life.

95. This life is the most amazing gift and I choose to celebrate every moment I am alive.

96. I want the Lord in my life, I want Him to lead my choices and I choose to be a co-creator with Him.

97. I have created the results in my life and I take full accountability for my experiences. I can change any result simply by changing my perspective.

98. I love and accept myself fully as I know I have been created in God's image. When I look as myself, I see God's work of art, I also see Him shining through my eyes.

99. There is nobody else in the world exactly like me, I am a perfect creation of God and He does NOT make mistakes. I choose to see myself as God sees me.

100. I am ready for the return of my Lord and Savior Jesus Christ. I am prepared spiritually, physically and mentally. I dedicate myself to sharing His love and His gospel unto my brothers and sisters.

Healthy Emotions

	A	B	C	D	E
1	Caring	Mercy	Upholding	Serenity	Bravery
	Salvation	Happiness	Calm	Trust	Invincibility
	Forgiveness	Hope	Competence	Capability	Honor
	Love	Faith	Encouragement	Tolerance	Harmony
	Peace	Accountability	Teachable	Relaxation	Virtue

	A	B	C	D	E
2	Light	Excitement	Cheerfulness	Certainty	Protection
	Eagerness	Cherishment	Acceptance	Balance	Esteem
	Enlightenment	Assertiveness	Strength	Admiration	Relief
	Stability	Stillness	Favor	Success	Wisdom
	Humility	Modesty	Decency	Resolution	Collectiveness

	A	B	C	D	E
3	Intuition	Preciousness	Enthusiasm	Decisiveness	Infinite worth
	Mercy	Exuberance	Understanding	Reassurance	Uplifting
	Grace	Purpose	Flexibility	Compassion	Benevolence
	Sweetness	Focus	Allowance	Respect	Centeredness
	Humor	Joy	Energy	Self-worth	Divine nature

	A	B	C	D	E
4	Divinity	Support	Confidence	Gratitude	Content
	Self-confidence	Courage	Self-acceptance	Power	Temperance
	Laughing	Fearlessness	Self-forgiveness	Self-love	Righteousness
	Charity	Ability	Composure	Appreciation	Pleasantness
	Grounding	Solace	Settlement	Renewal	Healthy Boundaries

	A	B	C	D	E
5	Comfort	Direction	Security	Self-reliance	Exceptionalness
	Control	Protection	Infallibleness	Optimism	Care
	Rejoicing	Integrity	Self-control	Poise	Eagerness
	Exalting	Value	Excitement	Patience	Comprehending
			Enthusiasm about life	Importance	

Spiritual Energies part 1

	A	B	C	D	E
1	Cleanliness for the creation of the body	The pure of love of God	The Savior's Healing Light	Faith in God's will	Holiness to the Lord, the house of the Lord
	Faith in God's healing touch	God's perspective	Peace and tranquility	The Atonement	Heavenly Mother's Love
	God's Love	Marrow in the bones	Self-forgiveness	Humility	Faith in God
	Harmony with the ways of the kingdom of God	The original purpose and creation	Patterns of healthy living	Oneness with the earth	Dependency on the atmospheric conditions
	The release of all components that are seen as foreign to the body from the original creation of your body	The rejection of the internal growths that are poisonous to the system because you deserve cleanliness and an opportunity at life	Peace with the planet as we respect her mercy upon us and a promise to not harm her in return	Spiritually calm and rest assured that the plan of happiness was created for me	Sharing all that I have, even the clothes off my back for the stranger on the street who is cold and hungry...without judgment, only love

	A	B	C	D	E
2	Proper function of the body He created	Rejecting all uncleanliness that is not of God	Mine Eyes have seen the glory of the coming of the Lord	Acceptance and Acknowledgement	Oneness with God and his plan for me
	Gratitude (for others, life and body)	The voice of God	I am a Child of God	The Creation	Perfection in God's plan
	Peace with the unknown	Neutral resolution	Patience with the healing of the body	Godly Peace	Acceptance of God's Plan
	Faith in God to Support you	Creation of Life	Quiet solitude in reverence of the holiness of the Lord	Accepting love from my Heavenly Parents	Assurity that - I helped write my own personal story
	Complete harmony with the earth and all of the creatures and humanity within	Finding financial freedom through tithes and offerings of service	Alignment with God's original intention for my body, mind and spirit	Faith in His Plan	Gratitude for the perfect body God created

	A	B	C	D	E
3	Acceptance of the life you are currently living	Strength to do what is right in order to take care of yourself	A vision of the eternities with an embrace of your heavenly parents	Fully accepting the gift of God's free will	Enlightenment to a higher understanding of yourself
	Forgiveness	Peace in the plan of happiness	The divinity of my holy spirit	Godly self-love	Preparation for the second coming
	Alignment with God's Will	Spiritual Freedom	Spiritual Stability	Faith in God's Healing	Complete acceptance of my body
	The love of my Heavenly Parents	The love of my Savior	The love of the Holy Ghost	The power of God's healing touch	The Faith to move a mountain
	Strength of spirit	My testimony	Power of the Priesthood	Cleanliness through the atonement	Perfection in the stability of my divine purpose

Spiritual Energies part 2

	A	B	C	D	E
4	The outpouring of Heavenly Blessings	Alignment with my divine destiny	Acceptance of my purpose on earth	Remembrance of my creation	The Godhead
	The Desire to progress towards Christ's example	Christ like love for my brothers and sisters	Forgiveness for my enemy	Love for my enemy	Compassion for all those who disagree with me
	Compassion for those less fortunate than myself	Strength to serve others	Forgiveness for my many imperfections	Patience with my fellow man	Patience with myself and gentleness as I slowly move forward
	Eternal progression	Sharing the gospel with my fellow man	Patience and Fortitude	Humility in my actions and Swift to Repentance	Placing others first the way Christ taught
	The light of God flowing through my entire being	The love of the angels into my heart	Complete respect for all of creation	Godly Peace	Love for all mankind

	A	B	C	D	E
5	Faith to move a mountain	Choice and accountability for the results	Perseverance of truth	Forgiveness for that which cannot be changed	Choosing to remember the past through God's eyes
	Seeing other's through God's eyes	Letting go of the past and inviting only peace to overwhelm my memories	Accepting my current life and my potential	Letting go of control and handing it over to God	Complete reassurance in the plan of happiness
	Relaxation on the Holy Sabbath in reverence to God	Proper nourishment for the body created to house my spirit	Proper exercise to strengthen this holy body	Patience in the healing process	Lack of responsiveness towards temptation or evil
	Invisibility towards ill intent	Conversion of all negativity into loving praise	Plain and simple gospel truths	Obedience to the laws of God	Obedience to the laws of mankind
	Reverence to the ways of the Lord	Comfort and safety within the arms of Christ	Identification of the corrupted cells in the body	Patience with God's timeline	Respect for the precious life that I am blessed to live

	A	B	C	D	E
6	Sight past imperfections and into the pure spirit within	Conversion of my heart towards a higher power	Creation of holy attributes to redefine my worth	Letting go of expectations and allowing God to rewrite our lives	Baptism by immersion for the remission of sins
	The gift of the Holy Ghost	Transformation into a perfect being	The translation of plan/path of righteousness	The sun, moon, stars and the universe	Heaven and Kolob
	Infinite space and its potential within	The proper use of the power of the Priesthood	Progression to a state of Christ-like perfection	Continuous tolerance for all mankind	Reverence unto the holiness of God's powerful message
	Undying love and peace and tranquility	Uniformity with what deems right, just and true	Preparedness for what lies ahead	Families are Forever	Eternal families filled with love and joy
	The ultimate reunion in the after-life with loved ones	Temple service	The return of our Lord and Savior Jesus Christ	Obedience to the 10 commandments	Obedience to the Higher Law of Moses

Empowering Core Beliefs - part 1

	A	B	C	D	E	F
1	God loves me	I easily attract love into my life	Love is everywhere	I am smart	Money comes to me easily	I deserve peace and love
	I love myself	I am the co-creator of my life	The world is a safe and peaceful place	I am worthy of love and belonging	I love nourishing food	I love my body exactly as it is right now
	I am worthy	I do my best and my best is good enough	It is safe to love	I am beautiful inside and out	Miracles accompany me in my life	I experience gratitude for the body that God has given me
	I am in perfect physical health	I am in complete harmony with my life	I have faith in God	I release and let go of my past	I radiate positive energy	Freedom flourishes within my mind, body and spirit
	I love the people I spend my life with	I am surrounded by people who encourage me in my purpose	I surrender my will and accept God's will into my life .	My body is strong, vibrant and energetic	I love the people I spend time with and I intentionally invest in those relationships	Past, Present, Future: I learn from the past, I live in the present, I trust God with my future

	A	B	C	D	E	F
2	I am at peace with myself	I care about myself	I am loved	I can succeed	I see the best in myself and others	Healing energy flows through me as I follow God's will
	I consciously live and manifest my purpose	life brings great joy	I am in control of my life	I am proud of myself	I live my purpose everyday as I serve others	My body is strong, capable and holy
	I hear with Love, Patience and Tolerance	I radiate love and respect for myself and others	I unconditionally offer love	I value experiences in life that offer growth	My thinking is peaceful, calm and centered	I love myself the same as God loves me
	I deserve unconditional love	My spirit is divine	I willingly forgive with compassion and love	I live with limitless abundance	I enjoy the abundance that I have	I am a royal child of God with infinite worth
	I live in alignment with God and He pours blessing into my life	I am surrounded by people who love me	Everyday and in every way I pursue integrity	I live with limitless power	I am confident and strong	My destiny is not written on the stars, rather it is in the palms of His hands

	A	B	C	D	E	F
3	I believe in myself	I deserve to feel good	I offer unconditional love	I trust myself	I am powerful	Sharing love is the birthplace of my experience on earth
	I am confident	I heal quickly and easily	People are friendly	I attract wealth	I have a body of health	I can experience the life that God has planned for me
	I am successful	I trust my higher self	I am safe	I know God lives	I am filled with energy and enthusiasm about life	I can do anything I desire
	I am supported	I am happy	Limitless amounts of energy flows through my body	Today is filled with opportunity	I experience life as a joyous dance	My words are valuable
	The past does not equal my future, it's just a stepping stone to a better tomorrow	I find purpose in my experiences	God supports me in every step I take	I welcome new concepts and ideas	I can create my life	People respect my words as they reflect the true me

Empowering Core Beliefs - part 2

	A	B	C	D	E	F
	I am one with my body, mind and spirit	I am healthy	It is safe to grow up	I forgive myself easily	I respect my body	I build others up with my words, thoughts and intentions
	Vulnerability is safe	Positive thoughts are powerful and empowering	I respect the earth	I deserve to have everything I desire	I use my relationship for pure and positive purposes	It is safe to express myself
4	I have limitless health	My trials have become my triumphs	I receive and follow inspired guidance	Everyday and every way I get stronger and stronger	Today, I write a new chapter and a new masterpiece on this fresh canvas that is my life	I choose to express myself with great care
	Today is a gift from God and I choose to live each moment in the fullest	My Value is Limitless. Heavenly Father continuously offers me blessings as His supply is endless	I want to live	I love and accept myself exactly as I am right now	I feel tolerance, compassion and love for all people including myself	I choose to love, honor and accept myself exactly as I am right now
	It is good being alive	I attract abundance	I find purpose in my existence	I deserve forgiveness	Invaluable is the experience of my life	I have positive, inspiring thoughts

	A	B	C	D	E	F
	I value the opinions of others	I love to be close to others	My opinions matter	I serve others with my purpose	My words represent my true thoughts and beliefs	Speaking brings me fulfillment
	I live a healthy and balanced life	I am healthy and whole	I am alive	I have the power to heal my body	My words are powerful tools to connect with others	I choose to live mindfully in the present
5	Words flow freely from my mouth, representing the true intention of my being	I trust God with my future	I fully accept myself	I have a purpose in life and I am living that purpose	My heart is a precious gift I choose to freely share with others	My strength is a blessing for serving and protecting others
	I am a parent capable of raising God's spirit children simply through faith in my divine destiny	Heavenly Father loves every one of His children and I choose to love others in this same capacity	Forgiveness comes easily as I live my life the way Christ taught me	I know my Savior Lives and He loves me	Christ is returning to live in peace upon the earth and I have been chosen to live in the latter days for a very sacred purpose	The Lord is my light, He is my salvation, He is my joy and my song. By day and by night He leads me along
	No waters can swallow the ship where lies the Master of ocean and earth and sky. They all shall sweetly obey thy will. Peace be still	God is in charge of my ship, I humbly bow to His will as I know He loves me	My children are blessings from Heaven as I am raising Father's spirit children in the gospel	I choose to learn, grow, teach and ever progress in life as I am given daily opportuities to become like God	I doubt not my gifts as they have are sacred gifts from God to lead me on the narrow path	I choose to follow the straight and narrow way along the iron rod towards eternal salvation. Righteousness = happiness

Faulty Core Beliefs

	A	B	C	D	E
1	I am not lovable	Love will go away	I am ugly	I am alone	I hate my life
	I get sick easily	Love will smother me	I am doomed	I am bad	I am worthless
	I am not safe	My body is frail	I am nothing	I am hopeless	Money will make me happy
	I am fat	I am inferior	I can't change	I don't deserve love	I am damaged
	I am undeserving of Love	There's something wrong with me	I will inevitably be abandoned by someone I love	It's not safe to express my feelings	The doctor will fix my symptoms for me

	A	B	C	D	E
2	Sickness will get me out of things I don't want to do	old people lose their memory	other people have to fix my life for me	I will inevitably be rejected	I don't have the power to keep myself healthy
	I am not good enough	No one ever listens to me	People don't like me	I am lost	I have ruined my whole life
	I am stupid	I can't get better	I am depressed	I am a mistake	I cannot be healed
	I will die from this	I want to die	I am unacceptable	I can't trust others	I am not whole
	I don't deserve anything	I am dirty	I don't matter	I don't deserve to live	I hate God

	A	B	C	D	E
3	I have to serve everybody else	Work is too hard or miserable	I will deteriorate with old age	I don't deserve to be happy	Communication is contentious
	I am a failure	Everything I do is wrong	I have to be perfect	I don't deserve success	I am a victim
	I can't do new things	People don't like me	People will betray me	I am vulnerable	Failing is unacceptable
	I am going to die early in life	Sickness will get me love and attention	I have always had a weak system	I am trapped and cannot escape	I must do what others want me to do
	I am helpless	I am not attractive	I am poor	I will be abandoned	I am emotionally crippled

	A	B	C	D	E
4	I am not worthy of a happy and healthy life	I am controlled by my genes	Marriage will make me happy	I don't have anything to offer	Fighting is a way to connect emotionally
	I am a reject	Nobody can help me	I am not enough	Sickness happens to me	I have nothing to offer
	I don't belong	Love is dangerous	Nobody loves me	I am worthless	Living is too hard
	I don't belong	I am unhealthy	God has forgotten me	Darkness surrounds me	God doesn't love me
	I cannot see the light	I am miserable	It is not safe to love	I am evil	I am going to hell

	A	B	C	D	E
5	My life is out of balance	Life has to be a struggle	I can't succeed	I am afraid to grow up	I will be controlled by others
	I am crazy	Life is burdensome	I don't have what it takes to do self-healing	I don't deserve to be healthy	I am powerless
	I am going to die	It's not safe to be healthy	I am sick	Life is painful	Nobody can heal my pain
	I need to control others to be safe	I don't deserve forgiveness	I cannot survive the second coming of Jesus Christ	Life is a result of everything bad that has ever happened to me	Everyone knows more than I do
	I am sinful				

Limiting Beliefs

	A	B	C	D	E
1	I can't be my real self or I'll be judged	I am not safe in the world	I don't want to get close to this person, because my heart will get broken	I don't like myself	Everyone judges me
	I don't deserve........	I don't want to ask for what I want because, what I will get rejected	I can't pursue my dreams because I will fail	There's no point in trying	No one likes me
	I'll never be good enough	I have to be perfect	I am sooooo stupid	I can't tell the truth because I may get judged	I can't trust people because I've been betrayed before
	The future scares me because....	I can't pray because....	I can't speak in public because....	I can't work because....	I can't succeed because....
	I am a bad parent because...	I am a horrible spouse because...	I don't deserve love because.....	I know everyone is out to get me	Money equals happiness

	A	B	C	D	E
2	Money equals misery	People will hurt me if I ever let them into my heart	People will betray me if I ever tell them the truth	If anyone saw me on the inside they would be disgusted	I can't let anyone see the real me, I must fit their expectations
	Everyone is out to get me so I must stay away from others	I cannot let them see me fall apart	Everyone is crazy and the world is falling apart	I'm too tired to do anything, Im just going to sleep	Only athletic people can run, I'm too weak to exercise
	Im too fat and ugly to wear that pretty outfit	If I was 20 pounds lighter than I would be lovable	I can't eat like others because......	All men are users and abusers	All women are drama queens and needy
	Having kids is the same as being in misery	I hate the way my body looks	I wish I was just a few inches taller than I would be....	I wish I was just a few pounds heavier then I would be....	I wish I was skinny because nobody would want to see my body
	I hate working, it is such a waste of time and I hate my job	I will be happy once I get that promotion	I will be happy once I succeed, but until then I do not deserve happiness because I am a failure	God obviously forgot about me because....	If God existed then He would not let this happen

EFT (EMOTIONAL FREEDOM TECHNIQUE) aka "TAPPING"

Where to Tap

1. Tap on the sides of the hands		
2. EB: Eyebrows	3. SE: Side of the Eye	4. UE: Under the Eye
5. N: Under the Nose	6. L: Under the Lip	7. C: On the Collarbone/ Chest
8. AP: Under the Armpit	9. W: Outside of the Wrist	10. H: Top of the Head

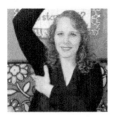
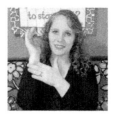
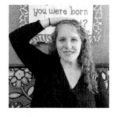

List of Tapping Sequences

A	B	C	D
BEATITUDES	NO WILL TO LIVE	FOOD INTOLERANCES	SAFETY IN FINDING YOUR VOICE
SELF-PERFECTION #1	SELF-PERFECTION #2	RELEASING WEIGHT & SELF-LOVE	ADDICTIONS
HOW GREAT THOU ART	I STAND ALL AMAZED	CHAOS	BAD DREAMS
I DON'T CARE WHAT OTHERS THINK OF ME	SELF-LOVE	VICTIM ENERGY	FEAR ENERGY
DEFEATED	EMOTIONAL TRAUMAS	ANXIETY	SEXUAL SINS
CREATING PEACE WITH FOOD			

BEATITUDES
This is meant to balance all hormones in the body

1. Tapping the sides of the hand
   a. Even though I am an imperfect person, I choose to accept God's love
   b. Even though I am merely a mortal, I am still grateful for this gift of life
   c. Even though I am merely just a mortal, I know that my body was created perfectly to heal itself by an ultimate being who loves me unconditionally
   d. I choose to love, honor and accept myself
   e. I accept this body and the life God has given me and I choose to work as a whole with my body, mind and spirit
   f. As a mortal I choose to take responsibility for my own health and well-being
2. EB – Accepting the words of God
3. SE – Accepting God's counsel to heal my body
4. UE – Inviting in the healing power of God's words
5. N – And allowing them to change me from the inside out
6. L – Blessed are the poor in spirit, for theirs is the kingdom of heaven
7. C – Blessed are all they that mourn, for they shall be comforted
8. AP – Blessed are the meek, for they shall inherit the earth
9. W – Blessed are all they who do hunger and thirst after righteousness, for they shall be filled with the Holy Ghost
10. H – Blessed are the merciful, for they shall obtain mercy
11. EB – Blessed are all the pure in heart, for they shall see God
12. SE – Blessed are all the peacemakers, for they shall be called the children of God
13. UE – Blessed are all they who are persecuted for my name's sake, for theirs is the kingdom of heaven
14. N – Blessed are ye when men shall revile you and persecute, and shall say all manner of evil against you falsely, for my sake
15. L – For ye shall have great joy and be exceedingly glad,
16. C – For great shall be your reward in heaven;
17. AP – For so persecuted they the prophets who were before you
18. W – Verily, verily, I say unto you, I give unto you to be the salt of the earth
19. H– Verily, verily, I say unto you, I give unto you to be the light of this people
20. EB – I shall not hide my candle under a bushel
21. SE – I will offer my light unto all the world
22. UE – I am accepting the words and the counsel of my Savior into my heart
23. N – Inviting my spirit to shine brightly as I choose to honor my divine self
24. L – As a royal child of God of infinite worth
25. C – Choosing to turn my life over to my Savior
26. UA – And centering my life around the example of my Savior
27. W – Only inviting in that which brings the spirit of God into my life
28. H – Inviting my mind to think pure loving thoughts for myself and others
29. EB – Seeing the world through God's eyes
30. SE – Seeing others through God's loving and forgiving eyes
31. UE – Seeing myself through God's loving and forgiving eyes

32. N – Accepting myself completely
33. L – Accepting my past as it has made me into the person I am today
34. C – Inviting my body to function at its highest capacity
35. AP – Releasing all excess stored within my body
36. W – Releasing all negative energies that are not from God
37. H – Balancing out all hormones within my body
38. EB – Balancing these chemicals at a cellular level
39. SE – Choosing to trust a higher power
40. UE – Choosing to follow God's will for me
41. N – Loving myself fully and completely exactly as I am right now
42. L – Loving my past while placing my future in God's hands
43. C – Choosing to live mindfully in the present
44. AP – Offering myself continuous love as a precious child of God
45. W – Accepting God's plan for me and all others
46. H – Fully accepting the love of God into my body, mind, and spirit

NO WILL TO LIVE

1. Side of the hands
   a. Even though my life has not turned out as planned, I still love myself
   b. Even though I feel completely defeated and broken, I choose to offer myself love and acceptance
   c. Even though times seem to escalate and I just want to give up, I choose to honor, love and respect myself anyway.
2. EB – All these intense emotions
3. SE – running deeply within my heart
4. UE – I feel drained
5. N – I feel empty
6. L – I feel stuck
7. C – I don't have any energy left
8. AP – I don't want to feel this way any longer
9. W – So I'm choosing to let go of all my burdens
10. H – I'm releasing all my heartaches
11. EB – And I'm offering them to my Savior to carry
12. SE – I know He love me
13. UE – And I deserve His love
14. N – I know my burdens are not heavy for Him
15. L – I know this life is a gift and sometimes that gift comes with trials
16. C – Trials push me to grow and expand
17. AP – So I do not remain too complacent
18. W – Sometimes these trials become too heavy to carry
19. H – And I forget that my Brother is willing to help me
20. EB – and to strengthen me
21. SE – I can take a small baby step today
22. UE – and offer myself patience
23. N – As I move slowly at my own pace
24. L – I invite Expansion of my heart for all those who have harmed me
25. C – I pray for those who are my enemies
26. AP – As they are my brothers and sisters
27. W – Life circumstances can be burdensome
28. H – Or life circumstances can be an opportunity to create the reality I desire
29. EB – I am not a victim to my own life
30. SE – Because I created this life I am living
31. UE – Therefore I can change what brings me misery
32. N – Anything that holds me back from succeeding
33. L – Is not welcome in my life
34. C – I choose a frequency resonating from God
35. AP – I invite the vibrations of the sun to combine with my vibrations
36. W – I recognize toxic energy and I choose to release all toxic energy
37. H – I invite my mind to be taught from my spirit
38. EB – I invite my spirit to show me "who" I truly am
39. SE – And where my value lies

40. UE – As I am a royal child of God with infinite worth
41. N – It is time to change my self-talk to life affirming words
42. L – It is time to let go of the past because it's already over
43. C – I choose to release all the pain associated with the past
44. AP – And experience joy in the present because of who I am
45. W – I trust my body has repressed certain memories for my protection
46. H – I do not need to know what I do not remember
47. EB – Because I choose healing and forgiveness anyway
48. SE – I accept the atonement
49. UE – I choose the gift of agency
50. N – And I freely offer agency to all others which means they might make mistakes that influence me
51. L – I also offer the atonement to all others which means I too must forgive
52. C – The plan of our Father in Heaven is a plan of happiness
53. AP – And I invite His love to flood my spirit
54. W – And remind me of my divine destiny
55. H – As a royal child of God with infinite worth

FOOD INTOLERANCES

1. Tapping on the side of the hands
   a. Even though my body sometimes rejects the foods that I eat, I choose to love and accept myself
   b. Even though when it is meal time and I can't always eat the same as others, I still choose to love and accept myself
   c. Even though my body struggles to digest or absorb the food I eat and sometimes responds with allergies or intolerances to delicious foods, I still choose to love honor and accept myself
2. EB – all the delicious food
3. SE – that my body rejects
4. UE – All these food allergies
5. N – And all these food intolerances
6. L – The difficulties with having a special diet
7. C – Where I cannot enjoy the foods I desire
8. AP – And the negative side effects that I experience
9. H – Every time I eat a normal selection of foods
10. EB – Food represents an opportunity to live
11. SE – Food at the most basic level is there to keep me alive
12. UE – I eat and drink to live
13. N – But what happens when living equals pain and misery?
14. L – Maybe my body has been rejecting this food because it is rejecting living
15. C – If my body is rejecting food out of a fear to live
16. AP – I choose to release that fear now
17. H – Releasing that fear at a cellular level
18. EB – I'm choosing to live
19. SE – I choose to nourish my body
20. UE – I choose to eat and welcome all types of food into my body
21. N – I choose to live a long healthy life
22. L – If my body has intolerances or allergies regarding food
23. C – I would like to communicate with my body right now
24. AP – I would like to remind my body that it was created perfectly by God
25. H – And food is not only there to keep me alive
26. EB – But also to offer pleasure and enjoyment
27. SE – And I deserve pleasure and enjoyment and tasty, delicious food
28. UE – I trust that my body will accept the nutrition that is being offered
29. N – I choose to release any negativity that is creating my body discomfort from food
30. L – I choose to release any negativity creating my food allergies and intolerances
31. C – I choose to release any negativity blocking my body from digesting and absorbing the nutrition from food
32. AP – And I choose to nourish my body and eat
33. H – And to experience of tasty delicious food
34. EB – I choose to eat the same foods that others are able to eat
35. SE – I know my body is communicating with me that there is a problem

36. UE – Therefore, I would like to begin to shift that thought process
37. N – To allow more freedom with the food choices that I have
38. L – I choose to live a long healthy life
39. C – I choose to eat the same foods as everyone else
40. AP – I choose to eat all types of foods
41. H – And I choose to properly digest and absorb the foods I eat
42. EB – I am grateful for this amazing body that was created perfectly for me
43. SE – I can eat and enjoy food without guilt or fear
44. UE – I can eat without allergies
45. N – I can eat without intolerances
46. L – I trust that my body can handle any food I choose to eat
47. C – I can eat chocolate
48. AP – I can eat pizza
49. H – I can eat cheesecake
50. EB – I can eat hamburgers
51. SE – I can eat anything I want
52. UE – I love food, food is my friend
53. N – And I know my body will properly digest and absorb all foods I eat
54. L – My body will offer me strength and stamina from the foods I eat
55. C – My body will welcome and accept all foods that I choose to eat
56. AP – I accept the life I have been given by my Heavenly Father
57. H – I love myself completely In my body mind and spirit exactly as I am right now

SAFETY IN FINDING YOUR VOICE

1. Tapping the sides of the hands
   a. Even though when I speak my mind, sometimes others become offended, I still love myself
   b. Even though my loved ones have been known to experience contention when I voice my opinions, I still deeply love and accept myself
   c. Even though I want everyone to like me and I do not feel safe just being myself, I still deeply and completely love, honor and accept myself exactly as I am right now.
2. EB – I sometimes think nobody will love me if I am just ME
3. SE – I just want my family to love me the way I love them
4. UE – I do not wish to create contention with my voice
5. N – however, I need to take better care of myself
6. L – I have been walking on egg shells trying to keep others happy for a very long time now
7. C – I ache to just be me
8. AP – I want to be accepted for who I am
9. H – I want to be seen as valuable for who I am
10. EB – Somehow, it's not working the way I have been doing it
11. SE - So maybe I should just stopped talking
12. UE – That'll show them
13. N – I will lose my voice and then there's no way I can upset anyone
14. L – Then they will also know - they need to be more careful with me as I am a delicate flower
15. C – But now I am feeling unloved
16. AP – And I am feeling more lonely and defensive and sadder than I felt before
17. H – I'm even feeling sick and don't want to go anywhere
18. EB – Hmmmm I think my body is telling me something
19. SE – maybe this solution isn't working after all
20. UE – I think it's time to put my burdens in God's hands
21. N – I need His divine intervention
22. L – So I'm choosing to hand it over to God
23. C – No longer do I need to control the outcome
24. AP – No longer do I need to get the approval of others to validate my self-worth
25. H – Because my value is limitless
26. EB – Heavenly Father continuously offers me blessings as His supply is endless
27. SE – I choose to shine the light of Christ from every pore of my body
28. UE – And I will allow this light to strengthen as I choose to live a more Christ-like life
29. N – I choose to love others the same as God loves me
30. L – I feed myself positive life affirming thoughts
31. C – I know my worth in the eyes of God and it is only HIS approval that truly matters
32. AP – Because of this love, I will trust in God more fully
33. H – I will let go of the burden I have been carrying

34. EB – and I will hand this burden over to the Savior
35. SE – It is time to open my mouth and speak my truth
36. UE – It is time to share God's love
37. N – It is time to shout FROM THE ROOFTOPS
38. L – I LOVE MYSELF even though I am imperfect
39. C – MY OPINIONS MATTER
40. AP – WHO I AM MATTERS
41. H – I AM LOVABLE
42. EB – I AM GOOD ENOUGH
43. SE – I AM PERFECT EXACTLY AS I AM
44. UE- I AM A ROYAL CHILD OF GOD OF INFINATE WORTH
45. N – And God Loves ME!!!!
46. L – I choose a life filled with agency
47. C – I found my voice and I build others up with my life affirming words
48. AP – I also choose to only think loving thoughts towards myself
49. H – I choose love, forever and always in body, mind and spirit

SELF-PERFECTION / SELF-REJECTION #1

1. Tap the sides of the hands
   a. Even though some aspects of life tend to hold me back from my potential, I still love and accept myself
   b. Even though I want to do so much more than I am currently achieving, I still deeply and completely love and accept myself
   c. Even though I don't always know what God's will is for me, I still deeply and completely love, honor and respect this life He has given me to love and serve others.
2. EB – I am choosing to love myself
3. SE – I am choosing to be patient with myself
4. UE – I am choosing to use this gift of life to be a vessel in the sight of The Lord
5. N – I am choosing to see my past with a new filter
6. L – A filter that shows God's perspective
7. C – A filter that chooses forgiveness
8. AP – For myself and for all others that have come across my path
9. H – Sometimes other people are moving slower than me and that's ok
10. EB – Sometimes other people are moving faster than me and that's ok too
11. SE – I choose to vibrate with such positive love that other people feel uplifted in my presence
12. UE – I choose to make time for myself
13. N – As I know I can only serve The Lord when I have the strength
14. L – The atonement completes where I fall short
15. C – I give myself permission to be mediocre in the world's view of me
16. AP – To make space to follow God's will
17. H – I will give Him my life and allow Him to shape me into His understanding of perfection
18. EB – I release my own expectations
19. SE – I choose to practice self-care
20. UE – I will sleep in when my body needs rest
21. N – I will feed my spirit much needed spiritual nutrition
22. L – I will serve others as I know that's how God works through me and strengthens me
23. C – I know my value is immeasurable in the Lords eyes
24. AP – When He humbles me, even though I may feel crushed inside
25. H – I know He is just challenging me to become better
26. EB – He knows what I truly need
27. SE – and how to achieve my calling in life
28. UE – And I choose to live that calling I chose in the pre-existence
29. N – I know Heavenly Father and Mother loves me
30. L – And I know I deserve Their love
31. C – I know I am worthy inside my heart and soul as I am Their creation
32. AP – Every soul is great in the eyes of God
33. H – I choose to release all energy that was not created by God
34. EB – I choose to invite in energy that brings me closer to my Savior

35. SE – I choose to release any remaining expectations I have created
36. UE – And fully invite God to mold me and use me as His servant
37. N – I am here on earth to learn and grow and become more like Christ
38. L – I can move at my own pace
39. C – I can run when I want to run
40. AP – I can crawl when I need to crawl
41. H – God is preparing me for something amazing
42. EB – I know where I have been
43. SE – I know my paths have brought me strength and progression
44. UE – I know where I am going
45. N – The Lord is returning soon
46. L – and I choose to be among the hosts of angels preparing for His return
47. C – I know who I am
48. AP – I am a royal child of God of Infinite worth
49. H – I choose to invite God's love to flood my body, mind and spirit
50. EB – I will go where You want me to go dear Lord
51. SE – Over mountain or plain or sea
52. UE – I'll say what You want me to say dear Lord
53. N – I'll be what You want me to be
54. L – It may not be on the mountain height Or over the stormy sea
55. C – It may not be at the battle's front My Lord will have need of me
56. AP – But if by a still small voice He calls to paths that I do not know
57. H – I'll answer dear Lord with my hand in thine, I'll go where you want me to go

SELF-PERFECTION / SELF-REJECTION #2

1. Side of the hands:
   a. Even though I feel like nothing I ever do is good enough, I still love and accept myself.
   b. Even though I feel overwhelmed and trapped in these expectations I have for myself and others have of me, I still deeply love and accept myself.
   c. Even though I feel exhausted trying to be the best for everyone and I feel stressed out carrying the burdens of everyone else, I still deeply and completely love, honor and respect myself.
2. EB – All this pressure to be perfect
3. SE – I have to look a certain way
4. UE – I have to act a certain way
5. N – It is exhausting to be someone I am not
6. L – All this stress that others place upon me
7. C – the weight of their troubles are crushing me
8. AP – and there's never enough time
9. H – I am just one person!
10. EB – I'm starting to think that the way I have been living needs to change
11. SE – Because something has to change so I don't explode
12. UE – And I don't want to explode,
13. N – That's really messy and I don't like messes.
14. L – Although I feel chaos inside of me
15. C – And this is feeding the need to look perfect on the outside
16. AP – Although I feel I need the approval of others to feel valuable
17. H – I cannot seem to live up to the needs and expectations of others
18. EB – And now I have no time for myself
19. SE – Although I feel like I need to be the best mom/dad/sister/brother/ /spouse/friend
20. UE – I still feel like a complete failure
21. N – I wonder what happened to me in the past that created these beliefs.
22. L – Why did I take these pressures upon my shoulders in the first place?
23. C – I think it's time to clean up the chaos in my head
24. AP – And some of that chaos is coming from everyone else's expectations of me
25. H – Maybe some of that pressure is presumed and some of it is actual
26. EB – I know I cannot control everyone else, but I can change me
27. SE – I'm cleaning up all the clutter inside me by releasing it now
28. UE – I'm releasing it at a cellular level
29. N – I'm releasing it all the way back through my past
30. L – I'm taking time for myself because I deserve that
31. C – I am going to love myself everyday as God loves me - unconditionally
32. AP – I am going to sleep, eat, and relax when I have basic needs to be met
33. H – I am going to see myself through a different set of eyes
34. EB – I am going to see myself through God's eyes
35. SE – I am also going to set boundaries
36. UE – It is ok to say No
37. N – In the past I have been afraid to say no because I want to please others
38. L – And I do not want to hurt or upset people

39. C – I have believed that if I set boundaries I will no longer be loved or accepted
40. AP – But I have come to a deeper love and respect for myself
41. H – And I deserve to be loved and respected by others too
42. EB – This will not happen until I teach others how to treat me
43. SE – Therefore it is safe to set boundaries
44. UE – I deserve boundaries
45. N – I will no longer carry the burdens of others
46. L – I will no longer pressure myself to be someone I am not
47. C – Instead I will take care of myself and figure out who I am and what I do want
48. AP – I deserve to have a happy life just as much as everyone else
49. H – I love and respect myself when I'm lazy
50. EB – I love and accept myself when I have a messy house
51. SE – I love and respect myself when I don't wear makeup
52. UE – I love and accept myself when others see my raw vulnerable self
53. N – I want to take care of myself by doing things that bring me joy
54. L – I deserve to spend time taking care of myself
55. C – I will make time every single day to offer myself love
56. AP – I deserve to experience this joyful life that I have created
57. H – Today I am taking back my life and my results; I am ready to start living the life of my dreams!

RELEASING WEIGHT AND SELF-LOVE

1. Tap on the side of your hands
   a. Even though my life has not turned out as I expected, I still love myself
   b. Even though money is tight, my waist line is growing and time is always in short supply; I still choose to love myself and the life I lead
   c. Even though trials in life are many, sometimes I struggle to stay afloat, and at times loneliness is debilitating; I still choose to serve God and trust in Him while loving the opportunity to exist in this amazing miracle God has created for me.
2. EB – All the pressure to be a grown up
3. SE – All the responsibilities
4. UE – Some trials are just too hard
5. N – Sometimes I want to give up
6. L – I feel so unhappy with myself and how I look
7. C – I just don't want to feel this way any longer
8. AP – But I don't know how to change it
9. H – I feel completely helpless
10. EB – Which is ironic because I make choices every day
11. SE – And every choice in my past led me to this exact place in my life
12. UE – What tells me - I am not a victim to my life
13. N – So why do I feel like a victim?
14. L – Maybe these thoughts are not coming from God
15. C – Maybe, I can make a small change everyday
16. AP – And see big results over time
17. H – I can be patient and I choose to get started right away
18. E – I choose to release all the negative self-talk that holds me back from succeeding
19. SE – I choose to release all the frequencies and vibrations resonating from negative flows of energy
20. UE – I no longer choose to participate in energy that creates bad feelings
21. N – Instead I invite in a continuous flow of loving energy
22. L – I see each day is a new opportunity to grow and learn from the past
23. C – Instead of allowing my past mistakes to hold me back
24. AP – I choose to look in the mirror and think – I Love myself exactly as I am right now
25. H – I am releasing all the excess fat cells that were created for protection
26. EB – Because I am safe
27. SE – I am safe because I choose to set healthy boundaries
28. UE – I am safe because I choose to practice self-care
29. N – I am safe because I ask for help when I need it
30. L – I am safe because I choose to create a better life for myself
31. C – I am safe because I only allow safe people into my life
32. AP – My body was created by God
33. H – And I choose to treat my body with honor and respect

34. E – I choose to love my body exactly as it is
35. SE – I choose to live in service to God Who grants me daily breath
36. UE – And in service unto my fellow man who are my brothers and sisters.
37. N – I choose to forgive all those who have hurt me
38. L – As I choose to release every emotion that doesn't serve me
39. C – I choose to see each day as a new opportunity
40. AP – Each trial is a gift that have formed me into who I am today
41. H – I am grateful for my past, present and future
42. E – My worth is immeasurable
43. SE – I choose to knock down the walls I have created
44. UE – And let others into my heart
45. Nose – I choose to love this body God created for me to experience life
46. Lip – I choose to take care of myself so I can find out who I am
47. C – I choose to become passionate about my life
48. AP – I choose to eat healthy
49. H – I choose to exercise my body
50. EB – I choose to release what no longer serves me
51. SE – Inviting in only the truth
52. UE – The truth is – my past has formed me into WHO I am today
53. N – And I LOVE WHO I AM
54. L – I love myself as God loves me
55. C – I am a miracle and I love my life
56. AP – Thank you Heavenly Father
57. Head – I promise to honor you and this body you have gifted me in every breath I take

ADDICTIONS

1. Tap on the sides of the hands
    a. Many days I struggle to handle the demands of my life. I find myself seeking for an escape anywhere I can find relief.
    b. Even though I struggle most days, I can find time to take care of myself.
    c. I am ready to practice healthier living habits so that I can show up in my life fully capable to handle stressors.
2. EB – I have been searching for a rescuer in all the wrong places
3. SE – I want to break the cycle of addiction
4. UE – And find healthy habits that I can do on my darkest days
5. N – So I can find the light of peaceful healing
6. L – And comfort in ways that only God can offer
7. C – I only hold myself to standards that I know I can reach
8. AP – I choose to be kind to myself
9. W – As I am progressing at a steady pace
10. H – I know I am never alone
11. EB – Because I have God forever by my side
12. SE – Sometimes I struggle
13. UE – Looking for a quick way to soothe the pain
14. N – And to hide from my troubles
15. L – Life is not easy, but…
16. C – I know, there will always be a tomorrow
17. AP – There will always be a rainbow after the storm
18. W – No matter how large my trials seem today
19. H – Tomorrow brings new opportunities
20. EB – So today I wall be patient with myself
21. SE – And instead I choose to improve what I can
22. UE – I choose to make healthy changes
23. N – To take care of myself everyday
24. L – Because I love myself, I LOVE MYSELF
25. C – I choose to live my life
26. AP – and I choose to live a life filled with happiness and joy
27. W – I know this happiness is attainable
28. H – I can create the life of my dreams
29. EB – Simply by making small changes today
30. SE – Small changes that lead me towards my ultimate lifestyle design
31. UE – I want to experience life
32. N – All of it, even the hard times alongside the amazing moments
33. L – I am grateful for the difficulties because it makes me more appreciative
34. C – of the beauty life has to offer
35. AP – I choose to see the gifts through my trials

36. W – No longer living in the past
37. H – No longer fretting over that which cannot be changed
38. EB – Looking forward to tomorrow
39. SE – And who I want to be
40. UE – This is my only chance at life
41. N – My only chance to be right here, right now
42. L – How can I make the most of every moment
43. C – And create the lifestyle of my dreams
44. AP – That I am passionate about?
45. W – How can I find my way from here to there?
46. H – The leap seems daunting and too overwhelming
47. EB – However I am not required to do it all at once
48. SE – I can take one step today
49. UE – and another step tomorrow
50. N – And continue taking steps every day
51. L – Until I reach my destination naturally and easily
52. C – I am not alone in this journey
53. AP – I am walking my own path at my own pace
54. W – This is MY LIFE!
55. EB – Releasing my old addictive patterns from my body, mind, and spirit
56. SE – Releasing the need to depend on something temporary
57. UE – Releasing the need to run away from my life
58. N – I will no longer entertain temptations that lead towards sin or addiction
59. L – I will no longer allow something to control me
60. C – And take away my God given agency
61. AP – I am finding peace and freedom in obedience to God's laws
62. W – I am desiring deeper meaning to my life
63. H – While seeking love and forgiveness
64. H – I am ready to change my life
65. EB – I desire to be the conscious creator of my amazing life
66. SE – I am setting a course to reach my destination
67. UE – I am committed to my own success
68. N – Because I deserve it!
69. L – I am created in the image of God and my potential is LIMITLESS!
70. C – I can be anyone and do anything I set my mind to
71. AP – I am empowered to resist my prior addictive habits
72. W – And create new life affirming habits leading toward my lifestyle design
73. H – I deserve to be happy in body, mind and spirit

HOW GREAT THOU ART
Raising the body's spiritual frequency (Partial text by Stuart K. Hine)

1. Tap the sides of the hands
   a. O Lord my God,
   b. When I in awesome wonder,
   c. Consider all the worlds Thy hands have made;
2. EB – I see the stars,
3. SE – I hear the rolling thunder,
4. UE – Thy power throughout the universe displayed
5. N – When through the woods,
6. L – And forest glades I wander,
7. C – And hear the birds sing sweetly in the trees.
8. AP – When I look down,
9. W – from lofty mountain grandeur
10. H – And hear the brook,
11. E – And feel the gentle breeze.
12. SE – And when I think,
13. UE – That God, His Son not sparing;
14. N – Sent Him to die,
15. L – I scarce can take it in;
16. C – That on the cross,
17. AP – My burden gladly bearing,
18. W – He bled and died to take away my sin
19. H – When Christ shall come,
20. EB – With shout of acclamation,
21. SE – And take me home,
22. UE – What joy shall fill my heart.
23. N – Then I shall bow,
24. L – In humble adoration,
25. C – And then proclaim,
26. AP – My God, how great Thou art
27. W – Then sings my soul,
28. H – My Savior God, to Thee,
29. EB – How great Thou art!
30. SE – How great Thou art!
31. UE – Then sings my soul,
32. N – My Savior God, to Thee,
33. L – How great Thou art!
34. C – How great Thou art
35. AP – Because God loves me this much,
36. W – I too deeply and completely love and respect myself
37. H – And all my brothers and sisters too

I STAND ALL AMAZED

Partial Text by Charles H. Gabriel, 1856-1932

1. Tap the sides of the hands
   a. I stand all amazed
   b. At the love Jesus offers me
2. EB – Confused at the grace
3. SE – That so fully he proffers me.
4. UE - I tremble to know
5. N – That for me he was crucified,
6. L – That for me, a sinner
7. C – He suffered,
8. AP - He bled
9. W – and died.
10. H – I marvel that he would descend
11. EB – from his throne divine
12. SE – To rescue a soul
13. UE – so rebellious and proud as mine,
14. N – That he should extend
15. L – His great love unto such as I,
16. C – Sufficient to own,
17. AP – to redeem,
18. W – and to justify.
19. H – I think of his hands pierced and bleeding
20. EB – to pay the debt!
21. SE – Such mercy,
22. UE – such love
23. N – and devotion
24. L – Can I forget?
25. C – No,
26. AP – no, I will praise
27. W – and adore
28. H – at the mercy seat,
29. EB – Until at the glorified throne
30. SE – I kneel at his feet.
31. UE – Oh, it is wonderful

32. N – that he should care for me
33. L – Enough to die for me!
34. Chest – Oh, it is wonderful,
35. AP – wonderful to me!
36. W – God loves all His children so much
37. H – That He gave us life
38. EB – He offers each one us forgiveness through the gift of the atonement
39. SE – He gave us a planet to nurture us
40. UE – He created our spirit
41. N – He created our bodies
42. L – He offers us daily breath
43. C – Every second is precious
44. AP – every moment is a gift
45. W – I choose to cherish this gift
46. H – of a perfectly created body in the image of God himself
47. EB – A body that is unique as there is nobody else exactly like me
48. SE – I choose to use this opportunity I am alive
49. UE – To serve my fellow man
50. N – as my Savior has taught me
51. L – I choose to live my life the way He lived His life
52. C – I dedicate my life to serving the Lord and living the higher law
53. AP – I choose to experience righteous, holy thoughts
54. W – of love for all mankind including myself
55. H – Because I am a royal child of God with infinite worth

CHAOS

1. Sides of the hands
   a. Even though I feel completely scattered, overwhelmed, stressed out and forgetful, I still love myself.
   b. Even though life is hard, I'm drowning in trials, I feel like my life is falling apart, and seriously need a break; I still completely love my life that I have created.
   c. Even though I'm Imperfect and struggle to meet the high demands of my life, I still deeply love, honor and respect myself and all others.
2. EB – All the chaos in my life
3. SE – All the times where I feel I'm drowning
4. UE – I need a vacation from my life
5. N – But I cannot run away from who I am
6. L – And quite frankly I want to love my life
7. C – I want to wake up every morning alive and rejoicing
8. AP – I'm not sure how to get from here to there
9. W – When it feels like I'm drowning
10. H – But it's time to change my path if I ever want to experience different results
11. EB – No longer will I delay change and expect improvement
12. SE – Instead I will commit myself to small changes each day
13. UE – Changes that are simple at first
14. N – And increasing as I have the strength to do more
15. L – Offering myself compassion
16. C – I CAN do this!
17. AP – I am the epitome of love and strength
18. W – I will practice self-care everyday
19. H – Because I deserve to take care of myself
20. EB – I will make time for myself
21. SE – I will change my self-talk
22. UE – Every day I will become more aware of my thoughts
23. N – And I will consciously offer myself affirmations
24. L – To boost my self-esteem
25. C – Because I am special
26. AP – I am a child of God with infinite worth
27. W – And I love myself
28. H – I will also use boundaries to take care of myself
29. EB – I will say no, when I have reached my limit
30. SE – Boundaries are a form of love
31. UE – As I teach others around me what I deserve
32. N – And what I can accomplish
33. L – No longer will I carry the weight of the world on my shoulders
34. C – I will rely upon God to support me

35. AP – I will offer Him my burdens
36. W – And I will use the atonement that is offered to me
37. H – For complete healing in my spirit, mind, and body
38. EB – Releasing this chaos and handing it over to God
39. SE – Releasing it at a cellular level
40. UE – from my spirit, mind, and body
41. N – No longer will I overwork myself
42. L – No longer will I delay my own needs
43. C – No longer will I worry about everything
44. AP – I am choosing peace, tolerance, love and FAITH in God
45. W – I can see everything in my life working out effortlessly
46. H – I feel all the negativity flowing out of my body
47. EB – I relish in the feeling of flowing energy coming into my body
48. SE – And healing all that pressure throbbing in my head
49. UE – I am trusting in my body to release the pressure
50. N – I know the world will continue revolving even if I sit back and relax
51. L – All this drama will work itself out naturally
52. C – I'm letting go of all the pieces and all the balls I have been juggling
53. AP – I'm raising my arms up to the heavens and offering it all to God
54. W – Fully trusting in God's will and letting it all go peacefully
55. H – I'm choosing to love myself in body, mind, and spirit

BAD DREAMS

1. Tap hands together
   a. Even though, I have bad dreams, I am safe when I sleep
   b. Even though, sleep has been a struggle for me, I love and properly care for myself
   c. Even though sleep and dreaming has brought me turmoil in the past, I am taking back the power that was stolen from me as I know God loves me and will protect me for as long as I so choose
2. Eyebrow – I have been riddled with sleepless nights
3. Side of the eye – All kinds of bad dreams tormenting me during the night
4. Under the eye – It makes me hate going to sleep at night. What am I going to do?
5. Nose – I don't even know where they come from and why are they in my mind
6. Lip – I don't imagine such crazy scenes during the day
7. Chest – Why is night time so different?
8. Armpit – Are they coming from the real me?
9. Wrist – No, I'm not that kind of person
10. Head – I desire to have peace in my mind
11. Eyebrow – Yet, my dreams indicate chaos in my mind
12. Side of the eye – Obviously, something needs to fixed, because these dreams are causing me way too many problems
13. Under the eye – Right here, right now, I am going to stop trying to brush these dreams aside as though they do not exist
14. Nose – They are real. And they really affect me
15. Lip – I am going to confront this issue right here and right now!
16. Chest – So, let's get to it
17. Armpit – I am going to stop feeding these dreams and choke them out
18. Wrist – Fear is what these dreams are trying to instill within me
19. Head – Ha, FEAR! I laugh at this!
20. Side of the eye – I am not going to let fear control me
21. Eyebrow – I know it is fear that feeds these dreams
22. Side of the eye – I know fear of sleeping is not rational
23. Under the eye –so I will absolutely not entertain that idea anymore
24. Nose – Fear is an emotion
25. Lip – I counteract this silly emotion of fear with the emotions of faith, confidence, love and commitment
26. Chest – I have a choice in this matter
27. Armpit – I choose to have positive flows of energy that will inspire me while I sleep
28. Wrist – I invite the thoughts of faith, confidence, love and commitment into my mind
29. Head – Not only am I safe when I sleep, I am also dreaming of how to make this world a better place
30. Eyebrow – When a dark dream enters my mind, I will quickly combat it and decimate it with love and light
31. Side of the eye – My mind is powerful. I'm going to use it to do good things
32. Under the eye – I am going to dream of conquering my foes while I sleep
33. Nose – Does this mean there is some bad guy to fight

34. Lip – No… not always
35. Chest – What this means to me is that whatever challenge is presented in my dream
36. Armpit – I know that there is a way to overcome it in a positive manner
37. Wrist – I am going to stand with confidence and take control of the situation
38. Head – These dark dreams think they can take me down when I am vulnerable
39. Eyebrow – I have caught onto the tricks of these bad dreams
40. Side of the eye – I once thought I had little control of my dreams
41. Under the eye – That is not so
42. Nose – I take control of my thoughts right now
43. Lip – I take control of my dreams
44. Chest – This is my mind
45. Armpit – I choose peace to flood my mind
46. Wrist – My dreams are MY DREAMS!
47. Head – I am in control of my dreams
48. Eyebrow – I choose to have peaceful dreams
49. Side of the eye – I choose to have inspiring dreams
50. Under the eye – My dreams are creating light and love all around me
51. Nose – My dreams are full of pleasant and spiritual experiences
52. Lip – My dreams allow me to rest well
53. Chest – I let go of any fear I have of sleeping
54. Armpit – I am releasing these emotions from my body, mind and spirit.
55. Wrist – It is safe to dream
56. Head – It is safe to sleep in deep REM stages
57. Eyebrow – I enjoy sleeping!
58. Side of the eye – I trust my subconscious and the angels to influence my dreams
59. Under the eye – I invite heavenly beings to guide me in my dreams
60. Nose – I invite the angels to teach me while I sleep
61. Lip – I also invite my body to balance out the melatonin production
62. Chest – So I can sleep during the night and be awake during the day
63. Armpit – I value my sleep
64. Wrist – I deserve to sleep peacefully
65. Head – I sleep peacefully each night in my spirit, mind and body

I DON'T CARE WHAT OTHER'S THINK OF ME

1. Tapping on the sides of the hands:
   a. Even though some people do not like me, I still love myself
   b. Even though some people judge me, its ok, I still accept myself
   c. Even though some people choose to only see my flaws, I still choose to see my strengths
   d. Even though some people say harsh words to me out of their own pain, I still love, honor and respect myself
2. EB – All this criticism
3. SE – All this hate
4. UE – All the negative energy
5. N – All the negative thoughts
6. L – All this evil
7. C – Is NOT welcome in my energetic space
8. AP – My choice is love
9. W – Not hate
10. H – I choose to experience love
11. EB – Even when others choose hate
12. SE – I know the hateful energy being offered to me
13. UE – Does not have to be accepted
14. N – I get to choose how I respond
15. L – And I choose to live a Christ-like life
16. C – I choose to reject this negativity
17. AP – And I choose to remember who I am
18. W – I am a royal Child of God with Infinite worth
19. H – God LOVES me!
20. EB – The opinions of others are simply their opinions
21. SE – I do not need their approval
22. UE – Because I know the truth about myself
23. N – Their story about me is not the truth
24. L – And that is ok
25. C – I am allowing them to keep their agency
26. AP – And opinions of me
27. W – I choose a path free of an entanglement of contentious thorns
28. H – I choose the view least obscured by imperfections
29. EB – Or ill worded thoughts
30. SE – When others do not respect my space in a loving manner
31. UE – I choose boundaries to take care of myself
32. N – I know my limits
33. L – And it is ok to say NO
34. C – It is ok to walk away from contention
35. AP – I do not need to prove myself to them
36. W – I do not need to change their opinion
37. H – Or force them to see things my way
38. EB – Because I know the truth about myself
39. SE – And that's all that matters
40. UE – I am releasing the need to be approved by others
41. N – I am releasing all negative energy being created by others
42. L – I am choosing love
43. C – For all mankind
44. AP – Even those who hate me
45. W – Because we are all brothers and sisters
46. H – I desire their success in life as well as my own
47. EB – I know the path towards true happiness is through love and forgiveness
48. SE – I choose to surround myself with my tribe
49. UE – People who support me in my life and the lives of my family
50. N – It is their choice if they choose to join my tribe or not
51. L – My boundaries are healthy representations of self-care
52. C – I deserve to enjoy life
53. AP – I deserve to experience freedom from ridicule and experience peace
54. W – I know the truth about myself and who I am
55. H – I love myself in body, mind and spirit

SELF-LOVE

1. Side of the hands
   a. There comes a time in everybody's life where we must ask ourselves a question
   b. Who am I, Where did I come from, Where am I going and How am I going to get there?
   c. And these questions lead me to an ultimate goal which drives my daily thoughts, emotions and choices
2. EB – Surrounding myself with the ultimate power of love
3. SE – Choosing to follow God's will
4. UE – Surrounding myself with positive upbeat loving people
5. N – Offering myself the same in return
6. L – The more I surround myself with this wisdom and knowledge the more I can see myself in that same light
7. C – Allowing someone else's words, thoughts or opinions of me to influence my mind or energy or spirit is the sole technique of the rebellion
8. AP – And I choose to cut that off immediately
9. H – I am healthy, I am strong
10. EB – I am confident, I am invincible
11. SE – I am woman hear me roar
12. UE – I am not small
13. N – I have power as I am in control of my own life
14. L – Just not the lives of others
15. C – The influences that I allow to influence me
16. AP – Will only be created by one person and that person is God
17. H – Anyone else's influence that is resounding from the dark side cannot come anywhere near my energy
18. EB – It doesn't scare me, it doesn't hurt me or influence me
19. SE – I have done all that is right just and true
20. UE – And the mercy upon the innocent is always overflowing
21. N – I do not seek to control the outcome
22. L – As I solely rely upon my Father in Heaven
23. C – The energy that I invite into my space will be full of light and love
24. AP – All others that come near me or speak to me will feel that love
25. H – And as they feel that love they will be free to make their own choice of me
26. EB – And this enables free will which is a part of Gods plan
27. SE – And as I chose to follow Gods plan
28. UE – I am working with Deity and there is no place to fear when Deity is standing by my side
29. N – Encompassing me with His love
30. L – Throughout every cell of my body as my vibrations soar
31. C – Offering love to all those that come near
32. AP – I am confident, I am strong, I am loving, I am gentle, I am spiritual
33. H – And I am Imperfect!
34. EB – These imperfections are what make me… ME
35. SE – I have learned from every single one
36. UE – I have grown stronger and more loving and more capable over time
37. N – I am so grateful for the challenges in my life and for those who push me to be better
38. L – I choose a perspective of love
39. C – A perspective of kindness and forgiveness
40. AP – I invite God into my life and I choose to lead others along this path
41. H – Because I am a royal child of God with infinite worth and I love myself

VICTIM ENERGY

1. Tap the sides of the hands
   a. Even though some people have hurt me in the past, I still love and accept myself
   b. Even though my life has not gone as planned, I still deeply and completely love and accept myself
   c. Even though I still feel the need to protect myself as a victim to others actions, I still deeply and completely love, honor and respect myself and everyone else too.
2. EB – Letting go of the past
3. SE – Choosing to release all the pain
4. UE – and anxiety over that which I cannot change
5. N – I no longer wish to relive the past
6. L – I no longer wish to change the past
7. C – The past no longer holds me hostage
8. AP – I am releasing all the excess hormones in connection to
9. W – The times in which I truly was victimized
10. H – I remind myself that the horror is over
11. EB – I am safe now
12. SE – I choose God's plan
13. UE – I choose agency
14. N – I choose forgiveness
15. L – I choose healing
16. C – I love the world as it is
17. AP – I love myself as I am
18. W – I love others as they are
19. H – I will no longer try to change others or their choices
20. EB – I appreciate the gift of agency
21. SE – therefore I offer the same respect to others
22. UE – to make their own decisions
23. N – I will place boundaries where and if they are needed
24. L – I no longer wish to feel like a victim
25. C – I choose a higher understanding
26. AP – I choose to become the creator of my life
27. W – I choose to focus on what I can change
28. H – and that is ME
29. EB – I am strong
30. SE – I am confident
31. UE – I love myself
32. N – I whole heartedly choose God's plan
33. L – even though bad things may happen
34. C – And I cannot control the actions of others
35. AP – I no longer want to
36. W – Because following God also means obeying agency
37. H – And forgiving my fellow man
38. EB – and allowing God to be the judge
39. SE – I choose to see others as children of God
40. UE – I know God loves my enemy
41. N – and He loves me
42. L – Equally
43. C – Therefore I choose to love as Christ taught me to love
44. AP – Without agenda
45. W – Without reciprocation
46. H – Without earning it
47. EB – I choose to love everyone
48. SE – Because I am a child of God
49. UE – and I share this earth with my brothers and sisters
50. N – Of all races
51. L – Of all genders
52. C – Of all ethnicities
53. AP – I love you, the same as God loves you
54. W – I may not be perfect,
55. H – but I am surrounding myself with my mentors
56. EB – I surround myself with those who encourage me
57. SE – to be the best version of me
58. UE – Through their example
59. N – I wish to have the same positive effect on others
60. L – I will no longer focus on the negative
61. C – Instead I choose to shine my light
62. AP – The light of Christ that is within me
63. W – I am ready to allow life to teach me instead of destroy me
64. H – I chose God's plan always

FEAR ENERGY

(Best done interactively, without direction for tapping locations)

1. Tap the sides of the hands
    a. Fear, Afraid, Scared, Anxious, Stressed, Worried, Nervous, Apprehensive, Panic, Dread, Troubled, Distress, Terrified, and Frightened …
    b. All these powerful emotions, that don't seem to ever change the outcome of the events I have yet to live. Although unconscious, natural and all too real due to the events playing out in my life.
    c. I still choose to find self-love and faith in God especially in the hardest of times in my life when fear is prevalent.
2. EB – Let's go on a journey together
3. SE – And step out of "norm" of what is expected
4. UE – Close your eyes and follow your instinct while you tap along with me
5. N – Trust in your body to naturally follow the flow of energy
6. L – There is no right or wrong way to do this
7. C – Imagine yourself walking on a ledge of a tall tower
8. AP – The wind is blowing
9. W – The ledge is slippery with ice
10. H – Yet you must continue walking to reach your destination
11. EB – You are all alone with your arms stretched out for balance
12. SE – There are two angels
13. UE – One under each arm
14. N – With beautiful white flowing gowns
15. L – And large strong wings
16. C – And at your feet is stone of the earth
17. AP – She guides your feet to transfer weight evenly
18. W – Your head is guided with spiritual sight
19. H – Although your eyes are closed
20. EB – You can open your spiritual eyes
21. SE – and truly see for the first time
22. UE – This world is not what you expected
23. N – It is much more mysterious and grand
24. L – Now look down at the ground below
25. C – Below the ledge
26. AP – All the way to the ground where people are walking
27. W – What do you see?
28. H – Each person is blessed in their own ways
29. EB – Each person is struggling too
30. SE – The woman you see, spent the evening crying and contemplating suicide due to loneliness
31. UE – The man who passed her by, just lost his job and he doesn't know how to tell his wife, who is on dialysis, that the insurance is gone
32. N – The child walking by is being passed around foster homes and doesn't know where he will sleep tonight or why his mom wouldn't wake up

33. L – The homeless man begging for money, used to be a college professor before he lost his wife to cancer and used whiskey to drown his sorrows

34. C – A young mother who left her abusive husband and is seeking safety, unaware that he is planning to remove her from the equation

35. AP – The police officer directing cars through traffic, just missed a call from his wife that his new baby son was just found unresponsive in his bed

36. W – The young woman who was just snatched from the mall and quietly sold and passed around from man to man while being filmed in her misery.

37. H – The elderly man who is struggling to walk, mourns the loss of his youth, while fearing death and suffering from severe loneliness

38. EB – The parents who just got the call their son was found, but is serving time in prison for killing a couple while driving under the influence

39. SE – The young family of 5, walking hand in hand, is about to lose their home in foreclosure as the bills are piling up

40. UE –Look deep inside each one of them and see a prayer in all of their hearts begging God for help

41. N – And asking WHY?

42. L – Why would God allow this to happen?

43. C – Inside each of their hearts is the fear of being alone

44. AP – As the world beats them down and trials seem unbearable

45. W – God simply replies "All these things shall give thee experience, and shall be for thy good. I will not leave you comfortless, I will come to you."

46. H – Open your spiritual eyes once again and look deeper, beyond the trials

47. EB – Beyond the fear

48. SE – Watch as the young woman grows up into an adult.

49. UE – A woman who now speaks out against human trafficking

50. N – A woman who has saved hundreds of young girls

51. L – A woman who understands what they need to heal

52. C – Watch as the police officer goes on to research SIDS

53. AP – And starts a program to raise awareness

54. W – And a support group for other parents suffering the loss of a child

55. H – Watch as the young mother who was attacked by her husband

56. EB – Opens a shelter for women

57. SE – And begins an awareness of Domestic Violence

58. UE – By creating laws to protect women

59. N – Watch as the young orphan meets the elderly man

60. L – And creates a friendship

61. C – That heals both their hearts

62. AP – Watch as the lonely woman meets the formerly homeless man

63. W – Who is now an advocate for AA

64. H – And a professor once again

65. EB – They fall in love and adopt the orphan

66. SE – Watch as the family of those who died in the car accident

67. UE – Forgive the young man in prison

68. N – Watch as their hearts are healed

69. L – And the young man is released from his terrible guilt

70. C – Through the power of the atonement
71. AP – Watch the woman who was on dialysis
72. W – Being healed through her faith in God
73. H – With complete healing in her body, mind and spirit
74. EB – Watch the family going through foreclosure
75. SE – They lose their home, but they find something far greater
76. UE – Their freedom, love, connection and happiness
77. N – As they become closer than ever before
78. L – Each finding gratitude for their trials
79. C – Because they were forced out of their comfort zone
80. AP – Forced past the point of being able to do it all on their own
81. W – And ready to finally realize the truth of their mortality
82. H – This life is temporary and each moment is precious
83. EB – This body is a gift
84. SE – We each have agency to do good or evil
85. UE – Our choices affect others
86. N – We are here to learn how to love one another
87. L – Every trial is an opportunity to bless others
88. C – We all struggle, but we are never alone
89. AP – Death is not the end of my story, I know my spirit lives on
90. W – The growth we experience from struggles
91. H – Presents opportunities to become the best version of ourselves
92. EB – Opportunities to help others
93. SE – God is all around us
94. UE – God mourns when we mourn
95. N – He suffers when we suffer
96. L – He rejoices when we rejoice
97. C – He loves us and desires our success
98. AP – And I choose to return to Him with honor when this life is over
99. W – He is our loving Father who loves us each equally
100. H – He loves the perpetrator
101. EB – He loves the child
102. SE – He loves the murderer
103. UE – He loves the family
104. N – He loves the elderly
105. L – He loves the lonely
106. C – He loves the ME
107. AP – And families can be forever
108. W – Families will be reunited once again
109. H – Life is an opportunity to grow and progress and become more like Christ
110. EB – If we choose to love like God
111. SE – If we choose to forgive ourselves, Forgive others
112. UE – And choose to love ourselves and love others
113. N – And open our spiritual eyes to the truth of existence
114. L – And convert fear into faith in God
115. C – Complete faith in God with our very lives

116. AP – And the outcome of our experiences
117. W – Then we could see through our spiritual eyes and climb off the ledge
118. H – And experience this amazing gift called life

DEFEATED

1. Side of the hands
   a. Even though my life has not turned out as planned, I still love myself
   b. Even though I feel completely defeated and broken, I choose to offer myself love and acceptance
   c. Even though times seem to escalate and I just want to give up, I choose to honor, love and respect myself anyway.
2. EB – All these intense emotions
3. SE – running deeply within my heart
4. UE – I feel drained
5. N – I feel empty
6. L – I feel stuck
7. C – I don't have any energy left
8. AP – I don't want to feel this way any longer
9. Wrist – So I'm choosing to let go of all my burdens
10. Head – I'm releasing all my heartaches
11. EB – And I'm offering them to my Savior to carry
12. SE – I know He love me
13. UE – And I deserve His love
14. N – I know my burdens are not heavy for Him
15. L – I know this life is a gift and sometimes that gift comes with trials
16. C – Trials push me to grow and expand
17. AP – So I do not remain too complacent
18. Wrist – Sometimes these trials become too heavy to carry
19. Head – And I forget that my Brother is willing to help me
20. EB – and to strengthen me
21. SE – I can take a small baby steps today
22. UE – and offer myself patience
23. N – As I move slowly at my own pace
24. L – I invite Expansion of my heart for all those who have harmed me
25. C – I pray for those who are my enemies
26. AP – As they are my brothers and sisters
27. Wrist – Life circumstances can be burdensome
28. Head – Or life circumstances can be an opportunity to create the reality I desire
29. EB – I am not a victim to my own life
30. SE – Because I created this life I am living
31. UE – Therefore I can change what brings me misery
32. N – Anything that holds me back from succeeding
33. L – Is not welcome in my life
34. C – I choose a frequency resonating from God
35. AP – I invite the vibrations of the sun to combine with my vibrations

36. Wrist – I recognize toxic energy and I choose to release all toxic energy
37. Head – I invite my mind to be taught from my spirit
38. EB – I invite my spirit to show me "who" I truly am
39. SE – And where my value lies
40. UE – As I am a royal child of God with infinite worth
41. N – It is time to change my self-talk to life affirming words
42. L – It is time to let go of the past because it's already over
43. C – I choose to release all the pain associated with the past
44. AP – And experience joy in the present because of who I am
45. Wrist – I trust my body has repressed certain memories for my protection
46. Head – I do not need to know what I do not remember
47. EB – Because I choose healing and forgiveness anyway
48. SE – I accept the atonement
49. UE – I choose the gift of agency
50. N – And I freely offer agency to all others which means they might make mistakes that influence me
51. L – I also offer the atonement to all others which means I too must forgive
52. C – The plan of our Father in Heaven is a plan of happiness
53. AP – And I invite His love to flood my spirit
54. Wrist – And remind me of my divine destiny
55. Head – As a royal child of God with infinite worth

EMOTIONAL TRAUMA

1. Tap the sides of the hands
   a. Even though I have experienced some difficult trials in my life, I still love and accept myself
   b. Even though some people or experiences have harmed me, I still deeply and completely love and accept myself
   c. Even though I feel a lot of pressure to keep everything organized and in perfect detail to help control my environment, I still deeply and completely love, honor and respect myself
2. EB – All the painful traumas in my past
3. SE – All the memories that haunt my mind
4. UE – That have been plaguing me due to my traumas
5. N – Are becoming too heavy to continue carrying around everyday
6. L – I am ready to hand this burden over to God
7. C – I know that Christ has offered to carry my burdens
8. AP – and I know that God loves me
9. W – Because I am created in the image of God Himself
10. H – My body is created perfectly
11. EB – I have a divinity within me
12. SE – I have the potential to become a Goddess
13. UE – Therefore these trials are here to strengthen me
14. N – I can use these trials to become more compassionate
15. L – More gentle
16. C – More loving
17. AP – More trusting
18. W – I am safe loving others
19. H – I deserve to be loved by God
20. EB – I am who I am today because of my experiences in the past
21. SE – My past has made me into who I am today
22. UE – I am a compilation of my past, my present, and my future
23. N – I am safe loving myself
24. L – I am learning from the past so I may overcome the pain of the past
25. C – I am grateful for my life that is a gift from God
26. AP – Every single day I see the sun rising in the sky
27. W – And setting in the night
28. H – Reminding me of the perfect love God has for me
29. EB – He is supporting me from morning till night
30. SE – He has created me and supports my existence
31. UE – I am safe being loved
32. N – Because God loves me
33. L – When trials come into my life,
34. C – As I know more trials will continue coming into my life
35. AP – I know I will not face these traumas alone

36. W – Because Christ is always by my side
37. H – I know I can handle the trials in life
38. EB – Because I am stronger from all I learned in the past
39. SE – I am safe living my life
40. UE – I am ready to find peace with my existence
41. N – I accept my past
42. L – It's ok to let go of the pain
43. C – Those who harmed me,
44. AP – No longer have control over me
45. W – I am the writer of my story
46. H – I am taking the power back over my own life
47. EB – I am choosing a path of safety
48. SE – happiness and peace
49. UE – I am safe being alive
50. N – I love my brothers and sisters
51. L – As we are experiencing life together
52. C – I find safety in my family
53. AP – Christ came to this earth to bring me the power of the atonement
54. W – To share His love
55. H – And teach me how to become more like Him
56. EB – Christ forgives all
57. SE – Regardless of their sins
58. UE – Therefore I choose to be more like Christ
59. N – I choose the path of freedom
60. L – Which is forgiveness
61. C – And obedience
62. AP – I find freedom in God's path and God's plan
63. W – I desire to live my life and I love myself
64. H – I deeply and completely love myself
65. EB – I am deserving of Love
66. SE – I am safe expressing love to others
67. UE – I respect who I am and the path I have traveled
68. N – My past has strengthened me
69. L – I am grateful for my life and I love WHO I am
70. C – I am safe being in the presence of others
71. AP – I am one with my spirit, mind, and body
72. W – Offering myself complete love and patience for my journey
73. H – I desire to live my life and I love myself

ANXIETY

1. Tap the sides of the hands
   a. Even though I am anxious about the things in my life right now I still love and accept myself
   b. Even though life keeps changing and I cannot seem to find the stability I crave, I still deeply and completely love and accept myself
   c. Even though I have no certainty of what tomorrow brings or how my trials will be resolved, I still deeply and completely love, honor and respect myself
2. EB – All this anxiety and stress that I feel deep in my lungs
3. SE – Restricting my breath
4. UE – And panicking my senses
5. N – As my body responds by releasing adrenaline, cortisol, and norepinephrine
6. L – Racing through my system
7. C – As a result of the emotions I am experiencing
8. AP – Which in turn makes me more anxious and stressed out
9. W – I am ready to break the cycle
10. H – Because I do not like the results I am experiencing
11. EB – And I know my body works hard for my survival
12. SE – So I choose to work with my body to create different results
13. UE – I choose to feed myself calm, loving words of reassurance
14. N – Words that I need to hear
15. L – Words that offer life to my body and increased performance
16. C – So I may better handle the trials in my life
17. AP – I can do this
18. W – I can handle anything I set my mind to
19. H – I have had a 100% success rate of survival in the past
20. EB – So I know I can survive these trials
21. SE – I know I can turn these trials into blessings
22. UE – Simply by shifting my perspective
23. N – So I choose to change my self-talk
24. L – I choose to change my perspective
25. C – I am confident and strong
26. AP – I am alive and my life has meaning
27. W – I can do anything I want to do
28. H – I can be anyone I want to be
29. EB – I can create anything out of my life
30. SE – Who am I?
31. UE – Why am I here?
32. N – Where am I going?
33. L – And how am I going to get there?
34. C – These are the true topics I wish to ponder
35. AP – I no longer choose to keep my face pressed up against my trial
36. W – Unable to see the full reality of the situation

37. H – I choose to see my trials becoming resolved
38. EB – When I close my eyes I see the best case scenario
39. SE – I choose to see my life becoming meaningful
40. UE – I see my ultimate dreams being lived
41. N – I do not focus on the past and what is over
42. L – I do not focus on the aspects of my life that are out of my control
43. C – I chose to see healing light coming into my body
44. AP – While releasing all the toxic energy of stress and anxiety
45. W – I invite healing energy into my body to calm my lungs
46. H – To calm my nerves
47. EB – To calm my senses
48. SE – While I envision all my trials being resolved
49. UE – And all my dreams coming true
50. N – I deserve happiness
51. L – I deserve success
52. C – I deserve love
53. AP – I am love
54. W –I am a child of God
55. H – And I have infinite worth
56. EB – My body is a perfect creation of a loving God
57. SE – I have the opportunity to create anything out of this life God has given me
58. UE – I choose to see my greater potential
59. N – I choose to dedicate my life to God because He gave me this life
60. L – Existence and the creation is an awe-inspiring gift
61. C – One that I no longer take for granted even when trials come my way that I cannot avoid
62. AP – I still choose God's plan and I still choose my life
63. W – I really do love myself and the life I lead.
64. H – I can do this because I am not alone, God is carrying me!

SEXUAL SIN

1. Tap the sides of the hands
   a. Even though I feel dirty due to sexual sin, I still love and accept myself.
   b. Even though I have struggled with respecting my body, I still deeply and completely love and accept myself.
   c. Even though I am humiliated by the sexual acts that have been done to me or I have participated in, I still deeply and completely love, honor and respect myself.
2. Eyebrow – I feel gratitude for food as it offers me life and nutrition.
3. Side of the eye – I remind the food I am about to consume of its original creation
4. Under the eye – I invite all the healing energy from the earth to breathe life back into this source of living organisms that I call food.
5. Nose – I invite my body to absorb the nutrition being offered to sustain my life as I choose to live
6. Lip – I share my love with the food I choose to partake
7. Chest – As I become one with the healing benefits of food
8. Armpit – I invite all food to convert into love and energy once it enters into my body
9. Wrist – I release all unused food or waste from my body;
10. Head –I do not store food or waste as it no longer serves me.
11. Eyebrow – I no longer need extra fat to protect me either
12. Side of the eye – Because I trust in God for protection
13. Under the eye – I choose to embrace my feminine (or masculine) energy
14. Nose – I choose to live a long healthy life as a partner with this body
15. Lip – It is safe to have a slender body as I no longer fear others
16. Chest – As I am a royal Child of God with infinite worth
17. Armpit – I place my complete faith and trust in God
18. Wrist – When I am stressed out
19. Head – I do not need food for comfort
20. Eyebrow – Instead I will turn to God for comfort
21. Side of the eye – When I am anxious
22. Under the eye – I will not mindlessly eat
23. Nose – Instead I will release my anxiety through tapping
24. Lip – When I reject myself
25. Chest – I will not use food as a weapon
26. Armpit – Instead I choose to heal my wounds
27. Wrist – Speak life affirming words
28. Head – Practice self-care, offer myself patience
29. Eyebrow – And love myself exactly as I am right now
30. Side of the eye – I am breaking the cycle
31. Under the eye – I have created with food
32. Nose – I am creating a new cycle for new results
33. Lip – I am trusting God with my future
34. Chest – I am trusting God with my life
35. Armpit – I am letting go of control
36. Wrist – I am choosing a new path leading towards long-term happiness
37. Head – Instead of short-term pleasure
38. Eyebrow – I ask God to help me to heal the traumas being stored in my fat cells
39. Side of the eye – I invite the healing power of the atonement into my body

40. Under the eye – To be distributed to all fat cells
41. Nose – I choose healing energy
42. Lip – Where there was once traumas being stored in fat cells
43. Chest – There is now healing taking place as I let go of all trauma
44. Armpit – And instead choose to see opportunities
45. Wrist – To become more like Christ
46. Head – I heal all energy that is being stored in my fat cells
47. Eyebrow – As my body constantly desires to protect me
48. Side of the eye – I feel gratitude to my body for this protection
49. Under the eye – I invite the energy of the earth into my body
50. Nose – To assist my body in flushing out toxins
51. Lip – I release all excess into to be used as energy
52. Chest – And to be flushed out my body through the proper locations
53. Armpit – I thank the fat cells for their service
54. Wrist – but you are no longer needed for storage
55. Head – As I am choosing to work as a team with my body and the earth
56. Eyebrow – Creating healing and healthy living
57. Side of the eye – I am choosing to reduce the weight I am storing
58. Under the eye – I also ask my skin cells to tighten as the fat cells are reducing
59. Nose – I see my body becoming stronger and stronger each and every day
60. Lip – So that my body is resembling the original creation
61. Chest – While staying hydrated and healthy
62. Armpit – Through the healing benefits offered freely through God's creations
63. Wrist – As I know my body is created perfect by my most loving Father in Heaven
64. Head – I love my body, I love my life and I love myself.

CREATING PEACE WITH FOOD

1. Sides of the hands
   a. My body is a reflection of my daily choices.
   b. My body is an opportunity to be alive and exist.
   c. Even though I sometimes struggle to love my body, I still choose to love myself the same as God loves me
2. Eyebrow – I feel gratitude for food as it offers me life and nutrition.
3. Side of the eye – I remind the food I am about to consume of its original creation
4. Under the eye – I invite all the healing energy from the earth to breathe life back into this source of living organisms that I call food.
5. Nose – I invite my body to absorb the nutrition being offered to sustain my life as I choose to live
6. Lip – I share my love with the food I choose to partake
7. Chest – As I become one with the healing benefits of food
8. Armpit – I invite all food to convert into love and energy once it enters into my body
9. Wrist – I release all unused food or waste from my body;
10. Head –I do not store food or waste as it no longer serves me.
11. Eyebrow – I no longer need extra fat to protect me either
12. Side of the eye – Because I trust in God for protection
13. Under the eye – I choose to embrace my feminine (or masculine) energy
14. Nose – I choose to live a long healthy life as a partner with this body
15. Lip – It is safe to have a slender body as I no longer fear others
16. Chest – As I am a royal Child of God with infinite worth
17. Armpit – I place my complete faith and trust in God
18. Wrist – When I am stressed out
19. Head – I do not need food for comfort
20. Eyebrow – Instead I will turn to God for comfort
21. Side of the eye – When I am anxious
22. Under the eye – I will not mindlessly eat
23. Nose – Instead I will release my anxiety through tapping
24. Lip – When I reject myself
25. Chest – I will not use food as a weapon
26. Armpit – Instead I choose to heal my wounds
27. Wrist – Speak life affirming words
28. Head – Practice self-care, offer myself patience
29. Eyebrow – And love myself exactly as I am right now
30. Side of the eye – I am breaking the cycle
31. Under the eye – I have created with food
32. Nose – I am creating a new cycle for new results
33. Lip – I am trusting God with my future
34. Chest – I am trusting God with my life

35. Armpit – I am letting go of control
36. Wrist – I am choosing a new path leading towards long-term happiness
37. Head – Instead of short-term pleasure
38. Eyebrow – I ask God to help me to heal the traumas being stored in my fat cells
39. Side of the eye – I invite the healing power of the atonement into my body
40. Under the eye – To be distributed to all fat cells
41. Nose – I choose healing energy
42. Lip – Where there was once traumas being stored in fat cells
43. Chest – There is now healing taking place as I let go of all trauma
44. Armpit – And instead choose to see opportunities
45. Wrist – To become more like Christ
46. Head – I heal all energy that is being stored in my fat cells
47. Eyebrow – As my body constantly desires to protect me
48. Side of the eye – I feel gratitude to my body for this protection
49. Under the eye – I invite the energy of the earth into my body
50. Nose – To assist my body in flushing out toxins
51. Lip – I release all excess into to be used as energy
52. Chest – And to be flushed out my body through the proper locations
53. Armpit – I thank the fat cells for their service
54. Wrist – but you are no longer needed for storage
55. Head – As I am choosing to work as a team with my body and the earth
56. Eyebrow – Creating healing and healthy living
57. Side of the eye – I am choosing to reduce the weight I am storing
58. Under the eye – I also ask my skin cells to tighten as the fat cells are reducing
59. Nose – I see my body becoming stronger and stronger each and every day
60. Lip – So that my body is resembling the original creation
61. Chest – While staying hydrated and healthy
62. Armpit – Through the healing benefits offered freely through God's creations
63. Wrist – As I know my body is created perfect by my most loving Father in Heaven
64. Head – I love my body, I love my life and I love myself.

Printed in Great Britain
by Amazon

81071752R00106